With

The Handbook for Advanced Primary Care Nurses

CUSTOMER SERVI

The Handbook for Advanced Primary Care Nurses

Edited by
Rebecca Neno and Debby Price

 Open University Press

Open University Press
McGraw-Hill Education
McGraw-Hill House
Shoppenhangers Road
Maidenhead
Berkshire
England
SL6 2QL

email: enquiries@openup.co.uk
world wide web: www.openup.co.uk

and Two Penn Plaza, New York, NY 10121–2289, USA

First published 2008
Copyright © Rebecca Neno & Debby Price 2008

A catalogue record of this book is available from the British Library

ISBN–13: 978033522353-4 (pb)   978033522354-1 (hb)
ISBN–10: 033522353-2 (pb)   033522354-0 (hb)

Library of Congress Cataloguing-in-Publication Data
CIP data applied for

Typeset by YHT Ltd, London
Printed in the UK by Bell and Bain Ltd, Glasgow

The McGraw·Hill Companies

Contents

Foreword

Given the spectacular changes that have taken place within healthcare and nursing in the last decade and the direction of current health reform, I am delighted to write the foreword for this highly topical book. Its publication is timely given the times which nurses are working in – changes in disease patterns, a very different society from the one that existed at the time of the start of the NHS and rapid advances in technology and drug therapy. Working in a constantly evolving health setting is certainly challenging for nurses and also exciting, but for many, quite demanding and unsettling. Constant learning is essential and adapting to working well within a workforce that is different in style and form from the traditional one is a huge issue, but one that nurses should feel confident and competent to manage.

These are just some of the reasons why *The Handbook for Advanced Primary Care Nurses* is so necessary to the career development of talented nurses and will, without doubt, be welcomed by them. Newly qualified nurses embarking on their careers should also be introduced to this textbook. It is entirely appropriate that we have a new nursing book focusing on the many developments taking place – and that will continue to take place – in the community health setting. While, historically, the hospital nurse has been the centre of attention, in more recent years, politicians have driven a health agenda that aims to expand and enhance primary care. The significant aims and hopes being that, as a nation, we become better at preventing disease, improving health and healthcare services, while at the same time diminishing hospital demand.

Despite inevitable problems and difficulties, the opportunities for community nurses are set to flourish, but we need the best possible nursing literature to help make this happen in a public health- and patient-centred spirit. Nurses must think about improving their analytical skills, learn how to manage complex demands without personal anxiety and approach work demands with enlightened, bold thinking and action. This book is destined to be a valuable asset to nurses determined to improve the quality of lives of those people who need the very best of nursing to help make this worthy aspiration a reality.

It is not before time that primary care should take centre stage of our healthcare system. In the 19th century Florence Nightingale wished to see a time without hospitals: 'My view you know is that the ultimate destination of all nursing is the nursing of the sick in their own homes ... I look to the abolition of all hospitals and workhouse infirmaries. But it is no use to talk about the year 2000' (Baley, 1987). In 2007 nursing makes up 70% of the health workforce, perhaps making it the most important discipline to get right, in terms of selection, education, preparation, knowledge, skills and expertise. In our rapidly shifting modern world, nurses need to constantly challenge their practice, their decision making and their relationships with colleagues, patients and the public. I believe that *The Handbook for Advanced Primary Care Nurses* should be extensively read and that it will prove to be an essential resource for nurses striving to improve public health and patient care in the communities of today *and* tomorrow. It may, with political will and a skilled and determined workforce, enable Florence Nightingale's vision to come true.

Reference

Baley, M. (1987) *A History of the Queen's Nursing Institute.* London, Croom Helm.

Lynn Young, RN, DN, CPT, FRCGP (Hons)
Primary Health Care Adviser, Royal College of Nursing

Contributors

Editors

Rebecca Neno, MSc (Distinction), BSc (Hons), SPDN, NPrescriber, RN Dip HE, Cert Health Promotion, at the time of writing was Primary Care Development Lead Thames Valley University, London, and is now Community Services Team Manager, Lincolnshire Teaching Primary Care Trust and Visiting Senior Lecturer, University of Lincoln.

Debby Price, MSc, BSc (Hons), Dip HE Health Visiting, PGCEA, RGN, RHV, RM, is Head of School, Community Health and Social Care, Thames Valley University, London.

Authors

Julie Bliss, MSc, BSc, PGDE, RGN, DN, is Head of Post-registration Nursing, Florence Nightingale School of Nursing and Midwifery, Kings College, London.

Lucy Botting, MSc Advanced Nursing, RGN, DN, CPT, NPractitioner, NPrescriber, RNT, is Head of Provider Modernisation and Professional Development, West Sussex PCT.

Gill Collinson, MSc, BSc (Hons), RGN, is Development Consultant and Director Social Enterprise Support Centre and former Director, Centre for Development of Health Care Policy and Practice, University of Leeds.

Rosemary Cook, MSc, PGDip (Applied Social Research), RGN, PN Cert, is Director, The Queen's Nursing Institute.

Karen Elcock, MSc, PGDip, BSc, RN, RNT, Cert Ed(Fe), FHEA is Director of Clinical Practice, Practice Education Support Unit, Thames Valley University, Slough, Berkshire.

Deirdre Kelley-Patterson, FHEA, MA, BSc, PhD, is Head of Centre, Centre for the Study of Policy and Practice in Health and Social Care, Thames Valley University, London.

Sarah Lewis, PG Cert (Long-term Conditions), BA (Hons), SPDN, Independent Prescriber, RN Dip HE, is Community Matron, Cambridgeshire PCT.

Marcus Neno, PG Dip, BSc (Hons), RN Dip HE, is Complex Case Manager, Lincolnshire Teaching Primary Care Trust.

Ian Price, MSc, Bsc (Hons), RMN, is Professional Lead for Mental Health, Thames Valley University, London.

Virginia Radcliffe, BSc (Hons), SPDN, NPrescriber, RNT, RN, is Senior Lecturer, Community Nursing & Prescribing, Centre for Primary Health & Social Care, London Metropolitan University.

Paul Thomas, FRCGP, MD, is Professor, Thames Valley University and Clincal Director, Ealing Primary Care Trust, London.

Michael Tullett, MSc, RGN, RMN, PG Cert (Ed), is Care Centre Manager, Chiltern View, Brendan Care Home, Aylesbury, Buckinghamshire.

Introduction

'The National Health Service celebrates its sixtieth birthday (in 2008) and access to primary care is one of the underpinning principles of the NHS ... sixty years on we can be justly proud of our primary and community care services ... with more than 90% of all contacts with the NHS taking place outside of hospital (The Rt. Hon Alan Jonson, Secretary of State for Health, DH 2008)

Primary care has seen a plethora of developments since the change of government in 1997 and there has been a rapid shift of care delivery and investment from secondary to primary care. This climate has provided opportunities for nurses and other allied health professionals to be at the forefront of healthcare delivery. This has been demonstrated by the development of new roles and services. These new roles and services require nurses and other allied health professionals to advance their current practice and encompass innovative roles within new skills and knowledge frameworks. Thus a new breed of advanced primary care practitioners is emerging.

Healthcare is being delivered in an ever-changing environment where roles and boundaries are constantly being challenged. This has led to the requirement for advanced primary care nurses to develop effective leadership, management and mentorship skills to enable them to function at both operational and strategic levels across organisational boundaries. In addition, advanced primary care nurses are expected to develop advanced clinical skills and knowledge and be able to diagnose and prescribe. As the healthcare world continues to change and develop, advanced primary care practitioners should now be involved with the identification of need, commissioning of services and service redesign as well as developing business skills and having refined communication and negotiation skills.

This book focuses on the knowledge and key skills that practitioners require to work effectively at an advanced level within primary care. The text is aimed primarily at nurses but may be relevant for allied health professionals and others working within primary and community care settings. The content relevant to advanced practice and primary care are broadly applicable and the social policy, legislation and details of specific services are relevant to the United Kingdom.

It is intended that this book will enable practitioners to develop their knowledge and skills through the completion of reflection points found within most chapters. These are meant to be thought provoking, allowing readers to link theoretical concepts with their practice and ultimately improve the delivery of care.

The book is divided into five parts to assist the reader in navigating the text: *Part 1* sets the context for the book, it explores the background, historical perspectives and influences of advanced practice in primary care. It is designed to provide the foundation of the book; understanding the history and origins of elements of care and practice should assist practitioners in the mission of moving forward and developing practice further.

Part 2 focuses on enhancing care delivery, with chapters covering these issues:

- legal and ethical issues in advanced practice
- case finding
- case management
- first contact and complex needs assessment
- non-medical prescribing.

Part 3 focuses on strategic developing and helping practitioners understand the strategic components of their role and includes chapters on:

- developing whole systems thinking
- transformational leadership
- developing and sustaining the role of the advanced practitioner
- developing and sustaining professional partnerships
- from involvement to partnerships and beyond.

Part 4 explores future trends in advanced practice within primary care and ideas as to how nursing may develop (and, indeed, currently is developing) to address these trends. Chapters in this part cover:

- commissioning in health and social care
- social enterprise and business skills
- influencing and getting your message across.

Part 5 looks to the future and asks what advanced primary care nurses may expect from trends and developments.

The contributing authors of this book have considerable expertise of advanced practice within primary care at both operational and strategic levels. We would like to extend our thanks to all authors who have contributed to this book and have worked hard to ensure their chapters are robust and contemporary. As such we hope that this book will ultimately make a contribution to enhanced care and support for patients and assist in the further development of the role of the advanced primary care practitioner.

Reference

Department of Health (2008) Foreword In NHS Next Stage Review. Our vision for Primary and Community Care. London, DH.

Rebecca Neno and Debby Price

PART 1
CONTEXT

1 Emergence of the advanced primary care nurse

Rebecca Neno, Lucy Botting and Marcus Neno

Introduction

The emergence of the advanced primary care nurse practitioner has been slow in comparison to their emergence and significance within the Untied States of America. This, in part, has been influenced by the development of nursing as a profession within the United Kingdom and also the structure of the National Health Service. This chapter will chart the development of nursing as a profession and the development of primary care nursing from its roots to the present day. The chapter will identify the origins of advanced nurse practitioners within the United States of America and how they developed as an autonomous professional group within the United Kingdom. Alongside this, relevant policy developments will also be discussed and the opportunities created for advanced primary care nurses identified with suggestions for developments in the future highlighted and explored.

Early nursing developments

The development of care in the community and community nursing have separate histories but both have had an impact on the way in which primary care nursing is delivered and practised today. The origins of the community care debate started with the Mental Health Act 1959, which was concerned with those with mental health issues and those with learning disabilities who had previously been kept away from the community in institutions. In comparison, community care of the physically sick has a longer history that has its origins in a number of places. These were mainly informal arrangements beginning with the priest St Vincent DePaul (1580–1660). He not only undertook the task of caring from the poor, but encouraged his parishioners to do the same by organising them and defining their roles after they had visited a home (Allan and Jolley, 1982).

In 1840 the Deaconesses' movement of the Kaiserwerth pioneered the building of a hospital under the direction of Theodor and Frederick Fliedner. This had a perpetuating effect, which resulted in the setting up of numerous other hospitals and the extension of the service of caring for the sick in their own homes.

In the 19th century, Poor Law committees undertook the task of employing parish nurses to care for sick people in their own homes. This was seen as cheaper than transferring them to the workhouses. Those who were not classed as paupers were cared for by visiting charities and, in 1840, Elizabeth Fry set up an institution based on the concepts of the Deaconesses' movement of the Kaiserwerth. The aim was to introduce women of the upper classes to training to care for their own sick (Watson, 2001). The success of the this venture was limited by poor structure and unclear goals (Fraser, 1980).

The first primary care nurses

Some years earlier, in 1859, William Rathbone, a Liverpool merchant, philanthropist and later an MP, had employed a nurse, Mary Robinson, to nurse his wife at home during her final illness. After his wife's death, he retained Mary Robinson's services so that people in Liverpool who could not afford to pay for nursing would benefit from care in their own homes. Seeing the good that nursing in the home could do, William Rathbone and Florence Nightingale worked together to develop the service. When too few trained nurses could be found, Rathbone set up and funded a nursing school in Liverpool specifically to train nurses for the 18 'districts' of the city and so organised 'district nursing' began.

The late 19th and early 20th centuries saw major and rapid changes taking place in the developments within health and social care (Watson, 2001). Midwives were regulated in 1902 and the notification of births became compulsory and the National Insurance Act was launched in 1911. By the time the NHS was launched in 1948 other health professionals such as school nurses had been introduced into some authorities.

Health visiting developed out of the UK public health movement of the late 19th century (Dingwall, 1977). Although the Health Visitors' Association was founded in 1896, originally known as the Women's Sanitary Inspectors Association, it was not until 1915 that the government formally created the position of the health visitor. However, the idea can be traced back to Florence Nightingale, who worked to raise awareness of the effects that poor sanitation can have on health. As a result of concerns over the high infant mortality rate in east London, a health visiting service was established in 1907. The child death rate halved in Ilford, London, during 1910–1912 following the appointment of the first health visitor in the area. During this time health visitors primarily provided information and focused on hygiene awareness, such as teaching mothers to clean feeding equipment. Health visiting was accountable to medical officers of health until 1974 and did not become an exclusive nursing speciality until 1962 (Robinson, 1982).

From 1919 when state registration for nurses became a reality, although the national standard fluctuated, at least it was possible to differentiate between trained and untrained nurses and General Nursing Council registration became a prerequisite for starting courses such as district nursing and health visiting. Eventually, in 1981, the specialist practitioner qualification was introduced and the United Kingdom Central Council for Nurses, Midwives and Health Visitors (UKCC) required the recording of the qualification on the nursing, midwifery and health visiting register. This qualification is still offered today but there is an increasing trend of fewer places available and a decline in applications, despite the continued investment within primary care services. The future of the specialist practitioner award should be addressed in the current review of post-registration education conducted by the Department of Health (see Chapter 15 for further information).

Reviews of primary care nursing

The Cumberlege Report (DHSS, 1986) on neighbourhood nursing, was the first report to recommend far-reaching reforms of community nursing services and health needs were considered to be inclusive of the following five key areas:

1   older people
2   disabled people
3   the chronically sick
4   the terminally ill
5   preventive care.

Today these five key areas have seen considerable improvements, for example the publication of the National Service Framework for Older People (DH, 2001), the End of Life Care Programme led by the Department of Health (2003), the enhanced focus on public health and health promotion (DH, 2004a) and the recent increased emphasis on the management of long-term illness conditions (DH, 2005a).

The publication of the NHS and Community Care Act in 1990 identified a much clearer understanding of how the government wanted services to be structured and delivered. The act introduced a number of fundamental changes in the organisation and delivery of care with the internal market and contract culture introduced for the first time into the National Health Service. This was seen by many as a major political turning point, emphasising individualism as a key feature (Watson, 2001). This period led to a degree of unrest with many concerned that the NHS was moving away from its core principles. The focus of service was pointed at the acute sector and as such resources were aimed at hospitals rather than primary care. This led to many rebranding 'care in the community' as 'care by the community'. The introduction of the Patients' Charter (DH, 1991) and the emphasis on the central role of primary care in the NHS (DH, 1997) began the redefinition and redirection of the National Health Service. The 1997 election of a Labour government began a new era of primary care services and development and one which we are still redesigning and evaluating today.

Policy context

Following the election of the Labour government in 1997, radical changes have occurred within primary care services. The internal market was abandoned and NHS community trusts were abolished. They were replaced with primary care groups and, subsequently, primary care trusts (PCTs), whose aims were to establish local need and provide services to meet those needs. There has also been an explosion of national service frameworks and clinical guidance fuelled by an interest in evidenced-based practice and a standardisation of care across the country. The government introduced targets into most areas of the NHS, including the 4-hour maximum wait target in accident and emergency departments, the 17-week maximum wait for outpatient appointments and the introduction of the quality outcome framework (QOF) into general practices where extra money is available for those practices meeting certain targets.

The ways in which primary care services were delivered were also radically redesigned. General medical services (GMS) and personal medical services (PMS) schemes were developed allowing general practitioners more freedom and the requirement for individual practices to provide an out-of-hours service became the PCTs' responsibility. This resulted in the employment of many advanced nurse practitioners to staff out-of-hours services in some areas. Appropriately educated nurses were, after many years, able to prescribe some medications and this in recent years this has been extended to include all the British National Formulary, with the exception of some controlled drugs (although this is expected to change in the near future) (see Chapter 6 for further information).

In 2005 further radical changes were announced about the structure of primary care trusts, with the introduction of commissioning within the National Health Service which has fuelled fear and anxiety as well as opportunity and excitement. Primary care trusts were required to split into provider and commissioning functions. The commissioning arm of the primary care trust is responsible for conducting health needs analysis and commissioning services to fulfil health needs. There is no guarantee that the provider arm of the same PCT would be awarded these contracts and they would need to tender against other companies interested in providing the service ensuring contestability. There are further requirements that ensure that PCT provider services are operating at arms' length from the commissioning arm of the PCT (DH, 2005b). (See Chapter 12 for further information.)

These developments have provided nurses with many opportunities to develop their roles and services but these developments also place a responsibility on nurses to develop skills in other areas such as business management, commissioning and running a social enterprise. Advanced nurse practitioners are ideally placed to develop these skills and will find themselves using them more and more in future.

Development of advanced nurses

While nursing and nurse education remained quite static in the United Kingdom during the 1950s and 1960s, revolutionary developments were happening in the United States of America. Within the medical profession there had been an increase in specialisation during this time. This had led to a large number of physicians leaving primary care, creating a shortage of primary care physicians and leaving many areas, especially rural areas, understaffed. In 1965, the Medicare and Medicaid programmes provided healthcare coverage to low-income women, children, older people, and people with disabilities. The sudden availability of coverage increased the demand for expanded primary care services. Because physicians were unable to meet this demand, nurses 'stepped into the breach' (Medicare Payment Advisory Commission, 2002). Nursing leaders believed that nurses were qualified to expand their roles and meet the need.

Some nurses and physicians opposed the nurse practitioner model. Certain nursing leaders believed that nurse practitioners were no longer practising nursing, that the title was 'ambiguous and misleading' and that such training in primary care medicine would 'control and devour nursing education and practice' (Nichols, 1997). Despite this, nurse practitioners continued to grow in number and autonomy in response to an expanding need for accessible, cost-effective care (Division of Health Care Services and Institute of Medicine, 1983).

Emergence of the advanced nurse practitioner in the UK

It was not until the late 1980s and early 1990s that the concept of the advanced nurse practitioner travelled across the Atlantic. The first nurse practitioners worked predominately in primary care settings, such as GPs' surgeries and homeless projects. Similarly, the majority of nurse practitioners are employed within primary care today (Ball, 2006). The Royal College of Nursing (RCN) in 1992 provided the first education preparation for advanced nurse practitioners with 15 nurses graduating; this set the precedent for many more to follow.

The RCN (2008) now defines an advanced nurse practitioner as a registered nurse who has undertaken a specific course of study of at least first degree (honours level) and who:

- makes professional, autonomous decisions for which she or he is accountable
- receives patients with undifferentiated and undiagnosed problems and makes as assessment of their healthcare needs, based on highly developed nursing knowledge and skills, including skills not usually exercised by nurses, such as physical examination skills
- screens patients for disease risk factors and early signs of illness
- makes differential diagnosis using decision-making and problem-solving skills
- develops with the patient an ongoing nursing care plan for health, with the emphasis on preventive measures
- orders necessary investigations and provides treatment and care both individually and as part of a team and through referral to other agencies
- has a supporting role in helping people to manage and live with illness
- provides counselling and health education
- has the authority to admit and discharge patients from their caseload and refer patients to other healthcare providers as appropriate
- works collaboratively with other healthcare professionals and disciplines
- provides a leadership and consultancy function as required.

In tandem with the development of the role of the advanced nurse practitioner in the United Kingdom, in 1992 the United Kingdom Central Council for Nursing, Midwifery and Health Visiting (UKCC) produced *The Scope of Professional Practice* (UKCC, 1992). This framework allowed nursing staff, where appropriate, to extend their roles giving them more professional freedom to take on responsibilities aligned to their practice environment. Although nurse theorists had shunned the use of the medical model within nursing advocating a holistic nursing approach to care, a British survey found that all advanced nurse practitioners were largely involved in work previously considered the domain of medicine and working within a biomedical model framework (National Health Service Management Executive (NHSME), 1996).

To support this contextual change within the field of primary care the Department of Health (DH) produced the framework *Liberating the Talents* (DH, 2002). This document proposed practical support and guidance on education and training. It emphasised 10 key roles (see *Box 1.1*) and three core role functions for nurses: first contact, chronic disease management and health protection and prevention. The DH collaborated with the National Health Service University (NHSU) to develop a work-based education programme, pushing the boundaries of nursing beyond its traditional safety net. The programme *First Contact* offered patients an acute high-level assessment within the primary care setting by advanced-level nurses.

Box 1.1 Ten key roles for nurses

1 To order diagnostic investigations such as pathology test and x-rays
2 To make and receive referrals direct to, say, a therapist or pain consultant
3 To admit and discharge patients for specified conditions and within agreed protocols
4 To manage patient caseloads for, say, diabetes or rheumatology
5 To run clinics for, say, ophthalmology or dermatology
6 To prescribe medicines and treatments
7 To carry out a wide range of resuscitation procedures including defibrillation
8 To perform minor surgery and outpatient procedures
9 To triage patients using the latest IT to the most appropriate health professional
10 To take the lead in the way local health services are organised and the way in which they are run

(Department of Health, 2002)

Development of new advanced nursing roles

Advanced nursing roles within primary care have continued to grow in recent years. Since the introduction of the community matron role (DH, 2004b) and contestability within the field of primary care (DH, 2005b, 2006) the advanced nursing concept appears to have gathered greater momentum, with the Department of Health emphasising the need for primary care nurses to provide higher levels of assessment related to physical, mental and social needs in order that they may prevent unnecessary hospital admissions; reduce the length of stay of necessary hospital admissions; and improve patient outcomes and ability (DH, 2004b). As good practice guidance, the Modernisation Agency alongside Skills for Health have produced a further document entitled *Case Management Competencies Framework* defining both the skills and knowledge of this new breed of primary care practitioner. The document suggests this will mean working at a level commensurate with the advanced practice requirements set by the Nursing and Midwifery Council (NMC) (DH, 2005c).

There has been a plethora of interest in the development of nursing in the home, the management of long-term illness conditions and the prevention of hospital admissions; however, there has been less activity in relation to public health. Despite promises made in Choosing Health (DH, 2004a) little money has truly been invested within preventive care. However, this trend may soon change with an increased emphasis on prevention of ill health and the role of the public health nurse in recent months. The role of the public health nurse equates well with that of an advanced practitioner (Burley et al., 1997).

Indeed, Labonte (1986) asserts since health is primarily an outcome of socioeconomic structures, public health workers must become a moral voice in the struggle to end social inequality. In practice, many health visitors do indeed plead their clients' cases with, for example, housing departments. It follows that the advanced practitioner in health visiting, in order to advance practice, may have to become explicitly political to truly embrace the new public health model and an advocacy function in practice. The advanced health visitor should not only work with groups such as minority and feminist groups and trade unions but should also be critically analytical in charting out health implications of policy and change (Luker and Orr, 1992).

Summary

The context in which primary care is being delivered is constantly changing and will continue to change in the future. Similarly, the advancement of nursing has happened swiftly and nursing roles will continue to evolve in the future. We face a number of demands within the United Kingdom, including an ageing population, a decreasing younger population and an ageing workforce combined with significant public health challenges, such as obesity. In conjunction, the political context is constantly changing and evolving and boundaries relating to roles and expectations are shifting. As advanced primary care nurses we must ensure that we equip ourselves with the necessary knowledge and skills to be able to keep apace of change. Workforce planners have a hugely important job in coming years to ensure that the workforce of the future is able to respond and adapt to changes within society and to provide high-quality care to those in need as well as playing a pivotal role in the prevention of ill health. Those at the centre of this provision are advanced primary care nurses and therefore the need for such professionals is only going to grow in the future.

References

Allan, P. and Jolley, M. (1982) *Nursing, Midwifery and Health Visiting since 1900*, 2nd edn. London, Faber & Faber.

Ball, J. (2006) *Nurse Practitioners 2006 – the results of a survey of nurse practitioners conduced on behalf of the RCN Nurse Practitioner Association*. Hove, Employment Ltd UK.

Burley, S., Mitchell, E., Melling, K., Smith, M., Chilton, S. and Crumplin, C. (1997) *Contemporary Community Nursing*. London, Arnold.

Department of Health and Social Security (DHSS) (1986) *Neighbourhood Nursing* (The Cumberlege Report). London, HMSO.

Department of Health (DH) (1991) *The Patients' Charter*. London, The Stationery Office.

Department of Health (DH) (1997) *The New NHS: Modern, dependable*. London, The Stationery Office.

Department of Health (DH) (2001) *The National Service Framework for Older People*. London, DH.

Department of Health (DH) (2002) *Liberating the Talents: helping primary care trusts and nurses to deliver the NHS plan*. London, DH.

Department of Health (DH) (2003) *Building on the Best: choice, responsiveness and equity in the NHS*. London, DH.

Department of Health (DH) (2004a) *Choosing Health*. London, DH.

Department of Health (DH) (2004b) *Chief Nursing Officer's Bulletin*. London, DH.

Department of Health (DH) (2005a) *Supporting People with Long-term Conditions*. London, DH.

Department of Health (DH) (2005b) *Commissioning a Patient-led NHS*. London, DH.

Department of Health (DH) (2005c) *Case Management Competencies Framework*. London, DH.

Department of Health (DH) (2006) *Our Health, Our Care, Our Say*. London, DH.

Dingwall, R. (1977) Collectivism, regionalism and feminism: health visiting and British social policy 1850–1975. *Journal of Social Policy* 6, 3, 163–169.

Division of Health Care Services & Institute of Medicine (1983) *Nursing and Nursing Education: public policies and private actions*. Washington, DC, National Academy Press.

Fraser, D. (1980) *The Evolution of the British Welfare State*, 6th edn. Milton Keynes, Open University Press.

Labonte, R. (1986) Social inequality and health public policy, *Health Promotion* 1, 3, 341–351.

Luker, K. and Orr, J. (1992) *Health Visiting: towards community health nursing.* Oxford, Blackwell Scientific Publications.

Medicare Payment Advisory Commission (2002) *Report to the Congress: Medicare payment to advanced practice nurses and physician assistants.* Washington, DC, Medicare Payment Advisory Commission.

National Health Service Management Executive (1996) *The Development of Nursing and Health Visiting Roles in Clinical Practice.* Leeds, National Health Service Management Executive.

Nichols, B. L. (1997) Nurse practitioners: the American experience. *Wisconsin Medical Journal* 96, 6, 16–18.

Robinson, J. (1982) *An Evaluation of Health Visiting.* London, Council for the Education and Training of Health Visitors.

Royal College of Nursing (RCN) (2008) *Advanced Nurse Practitioners – an RCN guide to the advanced nurse practitioners role, competencies and programme accreditation.* London, RCN.

United Kingdom Central Council for Nurses, Midwives and Health Visitors (UKCC) (1992) *The Scope of Professional Practice.* London, UKCC.

Watson, N. (2001) Nursing in primary care: an introduction. In Watson, N. and Wilkinson, C. (eds) *Nursing in Primary Care: a handbook for Students.* Basingstoke, Palgrave.

PART 2
ENHANCING CARE DELIVERY

2 Legal and ethical issues in advanced practice

Michael Tullett

Introduction

From a practical perspective, legal aspects of nursing have focused on upholding the Nursing and Midwifery Council's *standards of conduct, performance and ethics* (2008) and working within the scope of local employment procedures. Both, of course, reflect the legal process and act to shape ongoing legislation, while at practitioner level these shorthand applications are found most beneficial. Since the turn of the 21st century there has been a constant flow of information relating to legislation in health and social care practice. There are currently 16 different areas of policy under review, ranging across organisational policy, human resources and training, freedom of information, performance and equality to name but a few. This reflects the nature of change within health and social care, a change that is 'fuelled by increasingly well-informed public expectations' and the erosion of 'blind trust' in professional expertise (Nolan et al., 2001). It goes some way to underpinning practitioners' acceptance of codes of professional conduct as the mainstay in identifying the legalities of care and allows them to focus on care activities. Whereas this does not condemn the nature of change as a publicly driven agenda it does place practitioners in the frontline, where dilemmas are frequently encountered.

Much has been written about quality-of-life issues, although there is little to define exactly what quality of life is (Bond and Corner, 2004) and public demands are felt by practitioners in their everyday working lives. Increasingly, tensions are felt with the recipients of care questioning actions justified by professional conduct. It is suggested the basis for this tension is twofold. First is access to resources, a recognised tension that is displayed in recent publications (DH, 2005a, 2006a, 2006b). The focus here is on the provision of personal choice. The second is further from the public eye and yet is the foundation of our health- and social care-related legal process and that is the determination of 'best interest' and correspondingly 'deprivation of liberty' (DH, 2006c; WHO, 2005). These two aspects need to be discussed to determine the extent to which ethics have informed decision making at policy level and how the advanced practitioner may utilise different frameworks, be informed by legislation and deal with ethical dilemmas in their everyday activities.

Legal issues and frameworks

Legislation is essentially about creating a fairer society where everyone can participate and has the opportunity to fulfil their potential. The World Health Organisation identifies among its key principles that it is 'the ultimate goal of health policy to achieve the full health potential of everyone' (WHO, 2005). It goes on to further encourage the process of participation as 'crucial for health development' and offers three core values:

- **equity**: the achievement of full health potential for all
- **solidarity**: the sense of collective responsibility according to his or her ability
- **participation**: of both individuals and organisations working to improve the quality of public health decision making (WHO, 2005).

It may be timely to propose a framework to support the development of legislation that includes these core values and those promoted by the UK government of preserving dignity, confidentiality and autonomy implied in recent policy documents (NHS (Wales) Act 2005; NHS (Scotland) Act 2000; DH, 2006b; updated 2006). It would be more complete with values addressing the respect for people's rights and the provision of sensitivity to specific needs and vulnerabilities (WHO, 2005) and may look like Figure 2.1.

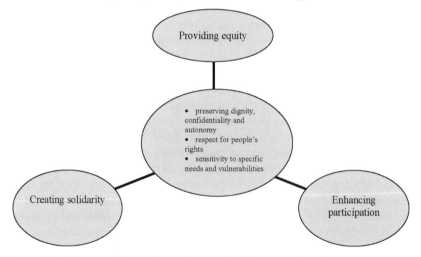

Figure 2.1 A framework for understanding the development of legislation

Given such a framework, it is worthwhile testing this against the basis for tensions including access to resources and the principle of best interest and deprivation of liberty.

In terms of resources, the Human Rights Act (1998) states both what your rights are under law and what you may say, do and believe. In relation to healthcare these include the right to life, liberty, respect for a private and family life and the right to be free of discrimination. Perhaps not so transparent are other rights that include to marry and have a family, freedom from torture and degradation, to education and to express oneself. Clearly, the framework accepts these rights, although, in practical terms, there are issues that arise.

In providing equity, there are judgements to be made surrounding the potential of the individual. This may be captured by the universal availability of resources, the universal accessibility of resources and the universal acceptability of such resources (WHO, 2005). Where resources exist and are accessible, the potential for an individual may be greater than in circumstances where resources are lacking or inaccessible. Equally, in some cases, resources are unacceptable (e.g. the acceptability of organ donation within deeply-held religious beliefs). On a grand scale these issues have been widely debated, but on a local scale the debate is frequently grounded in resource availability. Whether or not a patient receives a certain drug or type of dressing, has the services of a specialist or is generically supported is frequently controlled by what resources are fiscally available. At this point our framework becomes rhetoric. There is an ethical trade-off that amounts to equity versus cost effectiveness.

This may be relieved to some extent by the notion of solidarity. In this there is a sense of responsibility that includes all parties. Is it fair that one person should receive an expensive form of care in the knowledge that resources will be depleted for the next person? Is there not some personal sense of responsibility toward this 'next person'? These are questions relating to values. Where failure to supply resources will result in degradation or even loss of life for the sufferer, it fits with our societal and professional value systems to advocate for the patient and support all efforts to secure effective resources. It becomes a direct violation of human rights to withhold such treatment. However, not all circumstances are so clearcut. The WHO (2005) suggests it should be policy to ensure 'people benefit from scientific progress and its applications'. Where scientific and technological resources exist this may be interpreted as the right to achieve liberty and freedom from discrimination as the alternative of not receiving such support may be crippling illness and social stigmatisation. An example of such progress may be the development of new but costly pharmaceutical products. However, poor information systems and overriding organisational targets may make access to such resources a virtual impossibility. In this case, policy and service design may be seen to have resulted in an indirect violation of human rights. The question raised is where does solidarity start and where does it end? Within law there are a number of areas to consider. As a first line of action all people are entitled to an assessment to identify their needs. Where those needs are identified but not met there may be cause to bring this into the orbit of the Disability Discrimination Act (DDA) (Disability Rights Commission, 2005) which requires 'public bodies to promote equality of opportunity for disabled people'. Under the scrutiny of the Disability Equity Duty Agency, NHS and primary care trusts are to pay 'due regard' to the promotion of equality and are tasked to develop actions to improve services and information to disabled people and demonstrate such improvement over the next three years. The reality of this is any case brought before the courts under the DDA 2005 will require a substantial amount of evidence to identify what action was taken to improve the patient's life and what course this followed. Failure to do so will almost certainly result in a judgment against the trust. As a final recourse a person may then apply for hearing under the Human Rights Act 1998.

It is widely accepted that public participation is the answer to time-consuming and expensive legal battles. The Toronto Declaration makes it clear that organisations providing health and social care need to take a cultural perspective that facilitates such participation (Redfern and Ross, 2006). The WHO (2005) suggests 'both individuals and organisations [need to] work together to improve the quality of public health decision making'. In seeking to test enhancing participation (our third element of the framework), the issues fit around the difficulties encountered by people in exercising their right to act as full members of the community as a result of impairment.

Impairment itself is a complex socio-medical state and is closely linked to disability. Carol Thomas offers a model which recognises the power of the biomedical focus on the detection, avoidance, elimination treatment and classification of impairment (Thomas, 2002: 38–55). The outcome of such focus is to lead the sufferer into inevitable social difficulties and exclusion both as a causative factor (social perceptions of disability) and as a result of the impairment itself. The sufferer is somehow less of a person and 'lacks ability'.

The World Health Organisation endorsed the International Classification of Functioning, Disability and Health (ICF) with the primary aims of providing a scientific basis for consequences of health conditions, establishing a common language to improve communications, compare data on an international basis and provide a systematic coding scheme for health information systems, (WHO, 2001). Although Thomas (2002) argues that these models retain the biomedical element and despite a psychosocial element have little consequence to people with disabilities, the foundations of ICF are broadly speaking in support of conceptual transformation. The outcomes sought through scientific enquiry are those of human function, not merely disability, universal modality, rather than minority models alongside inclusivity and cultural applicability. This is would appear to raise people with impairments above that of a homogenous group and recognise the variants that exist, thereby offering more positive concepts to society at large. It is with this background that participation is called for on a legal basis. While fully supporting the call, there does need to be recognition of where the process is in real terms.

To assist this, Sapey et al. (2001) offer a helpful resumé of welfare enactments and disabled people, running from the National Assistance Act 1948 through the Chronically Sick and Disabled Persons Act 1970, to the National Health Service and Community Care Act 1990. In terms of participation it may be helpful to compare the language of the NAA 1948 (section 29) with current thinking:

> A local authority shall have the power to make arrangements for promoting the welfare of persons to whom this section applies, that is to say persons who are blind, deaf or dumb and other persons who are substantially and permanently handicapped by illness, injury or congenital deformity.
>
> (NAA, 1948: Section 29)

This section was later extended to include 'persons suffering mental disorder of any description'. This offers a paternalistic stance, although there was a change in the language used and the Community Care Act (1990) does start the debate around enablement and choice. However, the point underlined here is in demonstrating a system that valued doing things *to* people rather than *with* people and it is with this relatively recent history that society is trying to engage on a more equal basis with people who suffer impairment through illness. It is clear this element of the framework is in need of attention to assist this passage of change.

Case law and Mental Capacity Act

There have been a number of examples of case law, well documented in the past decade, and this chapter sets out three fairly well-known cases. Each may be described in the context of our framework. These are *R. v. North and East Devon Health Authority* (HSC 1999/180: LAC (99) 30, 11 August 1999) the Coughlan Judgment; *R. v. Bexley NHS Care Trust* (DH NHS Continuing Health Care, 25 January 2006) the Grogan Judgment; and *L. v. Bournewood Community and Mental Health Trust* (Misc (97) 84, 2 December 1997) the Bournewood Case.

The Coughlan judgment

Pamela Coughlan was seriously injured in a road traffic accident in 1971 and received NHS care in hospital until the closure of that hospital in 1993. The NHS moved care to a local provision, Marden House, on the basis this would be a home for life. In October 1998 the successor health authority decided to close this facility and transfer care to the local authority social services. Miss Coughlan and other residents challenged the decision on the basis the closure resulted in a breach of promise and was therefore unlawful. The challenge was successful for the residents of Marden House and resulted in far-reaching consequences in the way both the NHS and local authorities recognised and provided ongoing healthcare. Specifically, it was noted the NHS reached a decision that failed to meet statutory responsibilities under the Health Act (2006) and the criteria for providing such care were seen to fall short of its duty of care. Finally, the breach of promise constituted an abuse under Article 8 of the European Convention of Human Rights (1998) (Article 8 is the Right to Respect for Private and Family Life, Home and Correspondence (Human Rights Act, 1998)).

From a cross-agency perspective the case identified that agencies other than the NHS have responsibility for nursing care and local authorities may make arrangements to purchase nursing services. There was a requirement to clarify existing guidance, but it was lawful for local authorities to purchase services under section 21 of the National Assistance Act 1948. This did not mean the NHS no longer held responsibility where the person's primary need was for healthcare, but heralded new eligibility criteria for continuing healthcare and brought into being the NHS Funded Care (Registered Nurse Contribution to Care (RNCC)) (DH, 2001). This gave equity for those who required care and who had previously fallen through the net between healthcare and social care. It gave rise to a long and continuing discussion relating to the needs of people with long-term impairments, whose care needs, being beyond the influence of current medical approaches, were deemed to be socially based. The current eligibility criteria are set to identify those people who, because of the scale of their health needs, should be regarded as the whole responsibility of the NHS (NHS continuing care) while those who have fewer health needs may be supported by local authorities with some NHS responsibility retained (RNCC).

The Grogan judgment

The case of Maureen Grogan is less clearcut than that of Coughlan, in that there was no indication that the case brought to the courts was justified in terms of equity, but it does raise the interesting point of solidarity. Mrs Grogan was a widow with multiple sclerosis and suffered a number of chronic disabilities as a result of her illness. Following a fall she was admitted to a nursing home with the NHS accepting responsibility for medium-band RNCC. She argued her entitlement for NHS continuing care was denied as a result of the local trust using criteria contrary to the Coughlan judgment. The courts upheld the challenge on the basis the criteria used did not contain guidance regarding what tests or approaches were to be used while assessing the health needs of candidates.

The key points to arise from this judgment focused on the lack of clarity surrounding the interpretation of current guidance. Again the primary need should be considered as to whether or not this could be met by the local authority. It was considered inadequate that assessment should be uni-disciplinary and only through undertaking an holistic assessment of needs could the stability, complexity, predictability and risks be identified. Equally, the assessment process needed to establish first whether or not there was a primary healthcare need and only when this was clearly not the case should local authority responsibility have been considered. It was considered by the court that the NHS trust did not pay due regard to proving the needs of Mrs Grogan. This case identifies the demand in law to make resources available to meet the needs of individuals, as recognised by an effective, transparent and collaborative process.

The Bournewood case

This last case law scenario involves an autistic man who was informally admitted to a mental health hospital but who did not have the capacity to consent to such admission. Whereas there was no deliberation as to whether or not this man should have been admitted to hospital, the concern was in the process by which admission occurred. As such, the case demonstrates the demand for participation in our framework. Although based in mental health, this has concern to all in relation to people with cognitive impairment who are unable to consent to a specific form of treatment.

The implications are that any person admitted to a mental health establishment should have the capacity to consent to such admission or be held under section 2 or 3 of the Mental Health Act (MHA) 1983. Lack of dissent for admission is not sufficient cause for informal admission where there is lack of capacity. In the case of a person who lacks consent but is a danger to himself, it is acceptable to admit him as emergency, but satisfactory arrangements must be made for any continued detention. This case set a renewed focus on mental capacity and the way in which individuals should be partners in the process of care. A more detailed view of the Mental Capacity Act would be useful at this point.

Mental capacity is considered the normal value and any consideration of incapacity must be drawn from an acceptance the person is capable unless proven otherwise. Previous legislation in this area (MHA, 1983, Part 7) has been replaced by a new framework, to make it compatible with the European Convention on Human Rights (ECHR) Article 8. This new Mental Capacity Act received Royal Assent in 2005 and became law in October 2007. It consists of three parts focusing on (a) the person who lacks capacity, (b) a new superior court of record (Court of Protection) with new statutory officials and (c) technical provisions. The act extends only to England and Wales.

The starting point is a presumption of capacity and a support system that enables the person to make their own decisions as far as is practically possible. Decisions that appear unwise or against the person's best interest do not constitute reasons for applying lack of capacity. The reason for lacking capacity must be based in 'an impairment of or disturbance in the functioning of the mind or brain' (DH, 2005b).

Three features are required to determine a lack of capacity:

- the inability to comprehend information
- the inability to retain such information
- the inability to use the information, weigh it and arrive at a choice.

There is a fourth feature, rarely used, whereby an individual is in a 'locked-in syndrome', although this does not include people who are able to respond in a residual manner, for example, through blinking an eyelid to represent 'yes/no' answers. Action to support the safety and well-being of an individual who does lack capacity must be the 'least restrictive option' and must be least intrusive, 'interfering less with the rights and freedom of action of the person who lacks capacity' (DH, 2005b).

One key principle of the act is that all actions and decisions are taken in the person's best interest, although it is clear such a concept must be free from prejudice and stereotypical assumptions about the person and/or their circumstances. It is also incumbent on the decision maker to consider whether the person will have capacity at a later time and whether decisions may be held until this is achieved.

In taking decisions for another it is crucial to consider past and present wishes and feelings of the person. These may be identified through written statements, through recognising the person's cultural values, religious beliefs and past lifestyle choices and may be influenced by emotional bonds or family obligations. This information is most likely to be found in family, close friends or people who care for the person in a professional or voluntary capacity. In some cases a more formal representation may be found through an existing appointed advocate. The key principle in protecting decision making is found in the basis of 'reasonable belief', whereby decisions are made on the basis of substance. Where such substance is provided decision makers will not face civil liability. That said liability for negligence is not affected by this legislation.

Ethical issues and frameworks

At the start of this chapter two aspects were considered – access to resources, and the determination of 'best interest' and corresponding 'deprivation of liberty'.

In order to make valued decisions relating to care, there needs to be an acceptable framework on which decisions may be formulated and against which such decisions can be checked. The most commonly used ethical model is that described by Beauchamp and Childress (2001) in which the principles of autonomy, beneficence, nonmalificence and justice are demonstrated. This model has close associations with both medical and legal aspects of care and acts to underpin central themes of human rights in promoting autonomy as the primary principle on which actions are measured. Other principles may be overruled by the demand for autonomy, demonstrating the linear approach to the model. Based on Hippocratic principles, this has become the bioethical model of choice, but there are questions raised as to its adequacy in nursing. Different disciplines in health and social care may adopt different frameworks. Tschudin (1990) demonstrates this in describing the work of Gilligan whereby ethics need relativity to the work undertaken by a specific professional group.

A more recent work by Tschudin looks at the way in which ethics as a subject in nursing has changed over the past decade (Tschudin, 2006). She notes the increasing use of ethics as a way of developing coping skills based in the subject matter of philosophy and spirituality, demonstrating increased introspection on practice. In reviewing the publications of the *Journal of Nursing Ethics*, she claims ethical discussion has offered a forum through which previous poorly tolerated topics may be explored. This, in turn, has led to new understandings in care provision. This is very opportunistic as the issues relating to best interest and the deprivation of liberty have been in need of such exploration.

One such exploratory paper is that of Dudzinski and Shannon (2006). The approaches described accept the principle of autonomy as the key to life support measures. It is well accepted people have the right to refuse mechanical intervention or other forms of invasive medical support, but how this fits with the refusal of nursing care is a different matter. The authors describe a patient who is overweight and in pain. This patient experiences a host of disabilities that require some form of management in relation to incontinence and loss of mobility, but the patient has opted to refuse any further care as the pain experienced is too much to bear. Dudzinski and Shannon offer a number of approaches they describe as response measures.

In the first option, it is noted there is no paradigm within which to place refusal of care. In individual circumstances there is no consensus as to what care is necessary at what time and literature is forced to undertake a case-by-case review. Whether or not someone should accept pressure relief will depend on a number of individual factors. There is therefore no overarching approach to be taken in moral and ethical terms.

They note there are social taboos surrounding the refusal of care. The implications of a patient laying in excrement is both socially isolating and alienating to the individual and to the professional carer. It is more so where there are options to alleviate such a state and the professional carer is left to determine whether or not the refusal is a choice or an act of defiance. The consideration of best interest is a relative state that from a professional perspective may be influenced by the social taboo and by social norms.

Achieving a clean and functional state is a normal requirement for adults. In sickness, this role is to some extent undertaken by nurses and other healthcare professionals, but no matter who performs the tasks the state of normality remains. It is therefore antagonistic to normal social values to refuse these tasks being performed in the event of ill health and to do so results in carers experiencing a moral distress.

One way in which this may be relieved is described in the *autonomous response*. There is a need to determine the mental capacity of the individual, but that being confirmed there is no legal recourse for people providing care to insist care be accepted. It is suggested through undertaking an autonomous response the person's autonomy could be seen as relational. Rather than taking a purely action-based approach the autonomy of the individual may be upheld through negotiation and through providing respect throughout the care activity. Respect is demonstrated for the individual but the support offered for personal values and wishes does not prevent the care activity taking place. The ethical focus is on resolving the reason for refusal without reducing care activity. In terms of best interest there is no doubting the clarity of interpretation in such an approach, even though there may be doubt as to recognition of personal liberty.

An alternative approach is that of *conscientious objection* (Dudzinski and Shannon, 2006). It is recognised that professionals have the right to refuse to care for someone on moral grounds. However, this does raise the spectre of neglect and, it may be argued, merely passes the problem on to another. The main thrust of the outcome must be to actively seek alternative care should such objection be raised.

Closely aligned is the *communitarian response*. In this approach, the patient is considered in relation to the community in which he/she resides. Relationships, both personal and professional, form a part of this community and it is the good of the community that acts to drive processes. However, it is not clear where the criterion for such a drive originates. It would not, for example, be sufficient reason to insist someone is washed and changed just because of an offensive odour.

The next step along the path may be the *negotiated reliance response*. This is a proposed framework in which negotiations have a 'light touch' and the intention is to minimise distress of one's senses and sensitivities. There is minimal intervention and the intention is to develop a shared agenda.

The final approach presented by Dudzinski and Shannon (2006) is that of a *paternalistic response*, in which the notion of best interest overrides autonomy to protect the person from the negative consequences of refusal. The degree and role of negotiation in this response is to be considered, but if couched in the practised notion of informal consent, where care is apparently accepted through a lack of effective protest, it may be seen to be a common approach to achieving the expected level of care activity seen to be in the patient's best interest, although it could be argued that it fails to take account of the deprivation of liberty.

Where arguments of best interest occur they are frequently accompanied by ensuring ethical considerations are applied to avoiding exposure to excessive or unnecessary risk. The identification of risk often acts as the basis on which the relationships and communication processes develop between patients and professionals. Professionals hold status that provides an advantage in decision making within patient and professional interactions and it is argued that the concept of 'nurse knows best' remains something of a public perception. This concept in the establishment of 'best interest' is arrived at through analysing value-based judgements. This analysis is largely drawn from:

- making comparisons with other experiences
- clarifying key concepts in the approach to care
- developing a logical line of action.

Roach (1992) describes another framework she terms the 'five Cs', in which compassion, competence, confidence, conscience and commitment are the basis of developing ethical care. In these approaches, time is needed to take less of a linear view and more of a personal view that recognises the existence and the content of meaningful relationships in the person's life. The result of this perspective is the development of a logical response with steps that are drawn from the individual's account of illness and loss of well-being.

Consider and reflect on *Case study 2.1*, drawing upon the knowledge you have developed during this chapter.

Case study 2.1 Resorting to legislation

Peter retired from his construction business when decisions became difficult for him. He was diagnosed with Alzheimer's disease at the age of 56 and his wife and son have taken over the day-to-day running of the business. They keep Peter informed and seek his views.

Peter attends a day centre where he has recently been falling repeatedly. There have been a number of injuries and the district nurse attending produced a falls management plan. This has been difficult to implement as it entails that Peter reduce his activity considerably. The family are unhappy with the programme and identified a number of deficits:

- The programme is aimed at ensuring Peter does not fall on the day centre premises and has no application at home. The family believes it is intended to reduce corporate liability rather than meet Peter's needs.
- There has been no formal or medical assessment of the possible causes of his falling.
- Neither Peter nor the family has been involved in the development of the management plan but have been told it is the standard care plan developed within the PCT.
- The plan has acted to raise episodes of confrontation between Peter and the staff.

Peter fell and fractured his right arm during a struggle with a carer. The family are now in consultation with the legal profession to mount a legal challenge of neglect against the PCT and social services, which operates the day centre.

Reflection on case study

We work in a time where informed public expectations and increasing legislation, aimed to achieve full potential, have strong impact on our attitudes and behaviour. We need to adopt core values, equity, solidarity and participation but find dilemmas in equity arise where limited resources act to deplete the quality of care provision. Notions of solidarity arouse interest in the manner in which technical and scientific advances are developed and made available. If a treatment is developed but is too costly to purchase, or remains unrecognised by health and social care purchasers, it inflames public expectation and mocks the legislative process. Corporate information processes are important to advanced practitioners to enable client choice. Issues of equality are increasingly demanding clarity around the provision of information and promotion of choice. The information-giving process has to start with recognising difficulties that prevent the person with disability from exercising their right to achieving potential. In order to achieve this there needs to be acceptance of function being broader than that seen in an individual culture and from an individual 'well' perspective. Function is what can be achieved in an individual rather than a focus on preset socially-based limits as seen in welfare enactments of the past.

Lack of mental capacity may herald feelings of poor potential within individual clients and even in specific diagnoses. It is reasonable to suggest an advanced practitioner may recognise an inability to comprehend information and, in some cases, retain such information, especially in cases where the person suffers clear cognitive difficulties. However, the ability to use information, weigh it and arrive at a choice is not clearcut. Many practitioners will recognise the feeling of hopelessness in developing a certain approach, with the person being seen to be unable to cope with the decisions required. Where this is the case it is no longer acceptable to make such a decision without clear supporting evidence gained through an established assessment process that is aimed at achieving the individual's potential. This demands a strong emphasis be placed on collaboration with the person and those who are important to him.

Decision making is difficult where refusal of care presents. The social pressures felt by carers often dominate the outcome sought and the approach taken. It is worth reflecting the relationships that present in such cases and the coping mechanisms used by carers to resolve these difficulties.

Summary

Legal and ethical issues affect our professional decision making and without due consideration may lead to lesser care outcomes. This is recognised by leading authors in the field and Tschudin (2006) notes the positive impacts resulting from increased nurse engagement with ethical concepts in the past decade. The World Health Organisation (2005) offers three core values, equity, solidarity and participation, from which we may better understand and act within legal concepts underpinning our work. These core values have formed the basis of this chapter and it is noted that trade-offs inevitably occur in practice. This is a fact but should not diminish the goal of achieving these values wherever possible. Alongside resource difficulties many impediments to best care outcomes arise from the social construction of disability and impairment. These feature strongly in the case law scenarios, where equity, solidarity and participation were not solely resource dependent. New legislation arrives regularly and it is hoped that a focus on capacity is timely in providing some clarity around decision making where dilemmas exist. The focus on ethical approaches is a snapshot of some highly relevant work that has been undertaken in the past decade and is continuing unabated at this time. It is hoped the reader will engage fully with this work and develop a critical ethical approach to further develop the role of the advanced practitioner.

References

Beauchamp, T. and Childress, J. (2001) *Principles of Biomedical Ethics*, 5th edn. Oxford, Oxford University Press.

Bond, J. and Corner, L. (2004) *Quality of Life and Older People*. Buckingham, Open University Press.

Department of Health (DH) (2001) *Registered Nurse Contribution to Care*. http://www.dh.gov.uk/en/Policyandguidance/Organisationpolicy/IntegratedCare/NHSfundednursingcare/DH_4106715.

Department of Health (DH) (2005a) *Independence, Wellbeing and Choice*. London, DH.

Department of Health (DH) (2005b) *Explanatory Notes to the Mental Capacity*. London, DH.

Department of Health (DH) (2006a) *Valuing People, Moving Forward Together*. London, DH.

Department of Health (DH) (2006b) *Our Health, Our Care, Our Say*. London, DH.

Disability Rights Commission (2005) *Disability Discrimination Act*. London, DH.

Dudzinski, D. M. and Shannon, S. E. (2006) Competent patient's refusal of nursing care. *International Journal of Nursing Ethics* 13, 6, 608–621.

Human Rights Act (1998) *Public and Local Acts of the UK Parliament*. London, HMSO.

L. v. Bournewood Community and Mental Health Trust (Misc (97) 84, 2 December 1997) the Bournewood Case.

NHS Scotland (2006) *Delivering a Healthy Scotland Meeting the Challenge: health improvement in Scotland annual report*. http://www.show.scot.nhs.uk/.

NHS Wales (May 2005) *Designed for Life: creating a world class health and social service for Wales in the 21st century*. http://new.wales.gov.uk/docrepos/40382/dhss/reportsenglish/designed-life-e.pdf?lang=en.

Nolan, M., Davies, S. and Grant, G. (2001) *Working with Older People and their Families: key issues in policy and practice*. Buckingham, Open University Press.

Nursing and Midwifery Council (2008) The Code. Standards of Conduct, performance and ethnics for nurses and midwives. London, NMC.

R. v. Bexley NHS Care Trust (DH NHS Continuing Health Care, 25 January 2006) the Grogan Judgment.

R. v. North and East Devon Health Authority (HSC 1999/180: LAC (99) 30, 11 August 1999) the Coughlan Judgment.

Redfern, S. and Ross, F. (2006) *Nursing Older People*. Edinburgh, Churchill Livingstone.

Roach, M. S. (1992) The aim of philosophical enquiry in nursing: unity or diversity of thought? In Kickuchi, J. F. and Simmons, H. (eds) *Philosophical Enquiry in Nursing*. Newbury Park, CA, Sage.

Sapey, B., Stewart, J. and Harris, J. (2001) Disability: constructing dependency through social policy. In Baxter, C. (ed.) *Managing Diversity and Inequality in Health Care*. Edinburgh, Balliere Tindall.

Thomas, C. (2002) Disability theory. In Barnes, C., Oliver, M. and Barton, L. (eds) *Disability Studies Today*. Cambridge, Polity Press.

Tschudin, V. (1990) *Ethics in Nursing: the caring relationship*, 3rd edn. Oxford, Butterworth Heinemann.

Tschudin, V. (2006) How nursing ethics as a subject changes. An analysis of the first 11 years of publication of the *Journal of Nursing Ethics. Journal of Nursing Ethics* 13, 1, 65–85.

World Health Organisation (WHO) (2001) *International Classification of Functioning, Disability and Health (ICF)*. http://www.who.int/classifications/icf/en/.

World Health Organisation (WHO) (2005) *The Health for All Policy Framework for the WHO European Region*. Denmark, WHO.

3 Case finding

Michael Tullett

Introduction

Effective case management needs to identify and provide the support required for people with long-term conditions at an opportune moment along the patient journey (DH, 2005; NHS Modernisation Agency and Skills for Health, 2005a). To find those who need it we require rapid access to high-quality data. This forms the basis of this chapter – how do we identify and use data to identify care needs and, perhaps more fundamentally, does existing data and the systems that support care provision actually offer a lead in case finding?

Strategies for case finding

A vital step in developing a case-finding strategy is the development of a structured and systematic process that identifies the most vulnerable people taking account of the strengths of the existing infrastructure and current service provision. Case finding is the first step to providing early detection, good symptom control, effective medicines management and the promotion of user independence and self-control for people with long-term conditions. However, the current care paradigm is heavily influenced by the 19th-century notion of illness being a disruption of the normal state produced by a foreign presence or trauma. Traditional patterns of caring have acted to identify needs associated with disease management and efforts have been focused on meeting such needs through utilising available health and social service packages. The sum total of needs has not been recognised, resulting in fragmentation and care provision that has often been inadequate and incomplete (NHS Modernisation Agency and Skills for Health, 2005a).

With the increasing numbers of people suffering complex long-term conditions the political and economic focus is shifted from 'downstream' care (expensive acute-based) to 'upstream' (community-based) care, with the emphasis on the prevention of deterioration (NHS Modernisation Agency and Skills for Health, 2005b). In this context, case finding may be based on risk identification. The Predictive Risk Project clearly suggests 'PCTs should offer case management to individuals who are at "high risk" of an emergency admission' (NHS Modernisation Agency and Skills for Health, 2005b).

In support of this there has been a focus on designing systems of care provision such as Kaiser, Evercare and Pfizer, but less focus on the underpinning theories that broadly support such systems (University of Birmingham, 2006). Most literature takes a systematic approach to measure risk, using one of three main techniques. These are the *threshold approach*, where a threshold of acceptability is set and those who pass beyond the threshold are considered at risk (e.g. five hospital admissions in the previous 12 months); alternatively, risk is assumed through *clinical awareness*, perhaps seen in traditional approaches to care provision; and, third, through establishing a relationship between sets of variables, predictions of future risk are made. This last is the *predictive modelling* approach and is the major focus on case finding at this time.

There is less known around the prodromal phase of much chronic illness at the point whereby early intervention may reduce the need for costly medical interventions. There are two basic reasons behind this: first, the person needs to recognise that they have a condition that is susceptible to care; and, second, service providers need to respond to that recognition. It may also be argued that the main thrust of health policy has been placed on disease management, supporting the traditional clinical approach that starts from diagnosis, which in some cases may be very late in the course of illness. It has become clear there has been very little data on which to determine the needs of people at an early phase of long-term illness even to the point where they first enter the care system (King's Fund et al., 2006a).

Data management

At first sight it may be considered relatively easy to collect evidence about people who have been diagnosed or are receiving care, but the reality is that data management is not as advanced as could be desired. A number of approaches are used to extract evidence including prevalence surveys, detection and screening mechanisms, cohort studies/analysis and minimum datasets, to name just a few. However, these approaches need to be undertaken in populations that are diverse in terms of age, ethnicity and culture. To add to the complexity, attitudes to old age are frequently subject to misconceptions in relation to needs, beliefs and wishes, ethnicity is equally subject to loose preconceptions and the beliefs and expectations of people with long-term conditions are not widely understood in practice. Identifying and predicting the need for case management does need to take these factors into consideration and is therefore more than the development of a register of disease and illness within a given population.

From a 'hands-on' perspective it is fair to say that the main focus in the new role of case management is currently on developing the clinical skills required to support the patient. Assessment techniques have overridden the consideration of case finding and there has been little strategic work or even personal reflection on this as a necessary focus. In the main, advanced practitioners involved are aware of electronic case-finding tools (PARR 1 and 2, predictive modelling and high-intensity user management systems) but find a lack of rigour in accessing such tools. It has become an administrative role to access the data and to send such data through to the clinical area, but with changing structures, roles and responsibilities within NHS trusts, it is common data that is not collected or not disseminated in a timely fashion. In August 2007 one group of community matrons reported the last 'run of PARR' was in February 2007. This is clearly unreliable in the establishment of a caseload and does not add validity to big picture analysis. As a result many practitioners have opted for more pragmatic solutions to case finding.

A number of local strategies have been identified including the identification and follow-up of people on GP lists who are housebound. Some practitioners have established regular contact with the ambulance services, following up people who have required emergency treatments and many practitioners work closely with social service teams providing home care, through either the single assessment process or personal liaison. There has been a focus on people suffering specific disease or conditions such as diabetes or thalassaemia and less specifically on 'clinical hunch'. In this, practitioners apply their experience to identify patients who through their current and predicted health state are liable to become high-intensity users.

While this acts to boost case finding at the beginning of the new role it will not necessarily promote sustainability and may well result in workloads that are heavily weighted to high-intensity users. As case numbers increase it is suggested there will be a need for a broader range of case finding including those who are at a lower level of need. The benefits of such a range will be longer term but cost effective as the provision of support at this level will ensure users are less likely to graduate to higher need with such unpredictable and sometimes frightening speed. Equally benefits are found in maintaining care standards and ensuring practitioners are not overloaded. Many NHS trusts are seeking case numbers of 50–100 patients per practitioner (Berkshire West, Kensington & Chelsea and Ealing PCTs are examples), resulting in a need for managerial support in outlining the scope of case finding and in identifying how users enter and leave the caseload.

A brief survey using the Ovid database in July 2007 found 645 studies relating to case finding. The majority of these focused on prevalence of a specific disease or illness (diagnosed or undiagnosed) within a specified community, supporting the disease management approach. The criteria for these studies were based on the presence or absence of symptoms of illness within a population holding, or potentially holding, a diagnosis. Whereas such studies have resulted in an increased awareness and, in some cases, an increase in health activity around effective health management, there is less support for population-based surveys being viable for case finding. Many such studies mirrored existing statistical tables (Porter et al., 2006) and, where studies were not well targeted, the number of people to benefit from being identified (3.9% of the sample population; Sanders et al., 2005) resulted in high cost per person. There is evidence that well-targeted population surveys are more effective. The Ealing survey of glaucoma (Patel et al., 2006) resulted in a 58% increase in referrals for specialist support. However, the efficacy of general population-based approaches as a central strategy in case finding for advanced nurses has not been proven and the use of well-targeted studies demands resources most often out of reach for community nurse practitioners.

Detection and screening

Case finding may be closely linked to detection and screening although such links may also be quite ambivalent. Detection is finding disease or ill health, while screening is the search for disease in people without symptoms. Detection is dependent on seeking specific health variables (clinical signs) to identify the components (symptoms) of ill health. This is not optimal in informing care management, though, as other variables will need to be considered relating to the individual qualitative aspects of ill health such as the individual's health beliefs, wishes and circumstances of the person within a lifecourse perspective and the impact specific components of ill health have on the person (Ozer and Cilingiroglu, 2007). Although detection does form one aspect of case finding it is not ultimate and may need to be contextualised to assist care management. Vandevoorde et al. (2007) contextualise case-finding programmes within the process of detection – detection is an outcome of case finding, rather than a feature of the process. It could be argued this is a matter of where the process starts and as such epitomises the ambivalence surrounding case finding seen at practice level.

The approach of cohort studies/analysis does offer a number of critical factors to assist the development of a case-finding strategy. A cohort is described as a group of people who possess a common characteristic while a cohort analysis attempts to measure some characteristics from one or more cohorts at two or more points in time. As a research technique, this approach is found in longitudinal studies, but as a case-finding technique the application of the principles of cohort analysis may be adopted to support the local experience of the practitioner.

To clarify, take a group of people who are aged 55 years old and more and who have a diagnosis of COPD. This combination makes the cohort unique. Then consider a comparison group, people aged 55 years and over who *do not* have a diagnosis of COPD. If you add a secondary characteristic, for example, the frequency of hospital admissions, it may be compared across the two cohorts at one or more points in time. We may then analyse the characteristics of the two cohorts and determine which cohorts are most admitted to hospital (see Figure 3.1). Vandevoorde et al. (2007) operated this method as a research technique to identify the impact of smoking on the frequency of hospital admissions. In advanced nursing terms it may be argued the existing knowledge of the practitioner of their current caseload may inform a cohort analysis through comparing different sections of a nursing caseload to identify the most acute and needy cohorts in local practices.

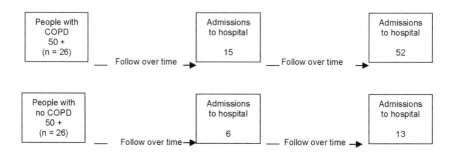

Figure 3.1 A cohort analysis (adapted from McCain, 2001)

This approach does prove frequent hospital episodes by diagnostic grouping, but does not identify individuals who require specific support. The approach leads to predictions about what conditions are likely to be most commonly admitted to hospital but does not provide the practitioner with a defined caseload. As a predictive model it is subject to the 80/20 rule (McCain, 2001), whereby 80% of resources will be used by 20% of the population. Figure 3.1 identifies hospital admissions in people over 50 years but other factors are crucial in the circumstances of hospital admission. Further work is required to take this raw data and clarify what the key factors (variables) are within the cohort and, if this is to be successful in reducing hospital admissions, what the components within the cohort are that may be altered to favourably impact on the course of care. This approach is termed *predictive modelling*.

Predictive modelling

Cohort analysis may therefore be used to develop a predictive model. Although it may appear similar, predictive modelling differs to screening processes. Repeated cohort analysis across the spectrum of diagnostic-led care provision will provide a rich database of conditions that have high impact on resource use. Such data may form the basis for a predictive model in identifying the key components that trigger higher levels of care. This is not specifically condition based but offers a broad approach to identify the key components of long-term conditions and the associated risks that are likely to result in hospital admissions. As such it moves beyond diagnostic categories and draws on common variables such as levels of deprivation, age, gender and/or occupation, alongside clinical data. These variables will assist in predicting what changes in care needs are likely to precede increased intervention across significant long-term conditions that are prevalent in the community.

There is good evidence to identify these common factors or variables, although where multiple long-term conditions co-exist this may be more complex. Early efforts to develop a predictive model focused on acute hospital episodes with the patients at risk of re-hospitalisation (PARR) (King's Fund et al., 2006b) being made available to NHS trusts from September 2005. The initial PARR used hospitalisation as a trigger event and algorithms included diagnostic information (so long as the diagnosis met with referenced conditions), patient characteristics (demographic data), the number and types of admissions over the past three years and the 'ward of residence'. This has subsequently been upgraded to identify a different 'trigger', being any emergency admission and does not rely on a 'referenced condition' but will identify any condition causing emergency admission (King's Fund et al., 2006b).

The baseline for predicting features (variables) of the PARR are:

- **Clinical conditions**: 32 most prevalent conditions offered initially. PARR 1 utilised specific identified conditions (a diagnostic subset termed *referenced condition*) but PARR 2 broadens the search to non-referenced conditions.
- **Patient characteristics**: demographic data of age, gender and ethnicity.
- **Ward characteristics**: community characteristics, cultural background, observed ration for MD practice, style, sensitivity.
- **Admission history** (prior utilisation): types and numbers of hospital admission and specialists seen.

At the strategic level, the intent is to predict the probability of service need in users over the next 12 months following identification, to improve health outcomes and to control health expenditure. Although a useful strategic mechanism, it is less helpful from a practitioner perspective where the ultimate intent will be to construct an illness trajectory with the aim of providing individualised proactive care management. The term *illness trajectory* was borrowed from physical sciences by Glaser and Strauss in 1968 to define the course of illness (Lubkin and Larsen, 2002). Over and above that information offered by PARR, a trajectory approach follows the path of illness including the actions taken by the patient and significant others. Through using such an approach practitioners may plot predicted needs in terms of phases of illness requiring self-management, service management, decision making and clinical intervention or support.

Lubkin and Larsen (2002: 10–16) identify the important predicting features as:

- **Growth and development factors**: biological, cognitive and social factors that are age related.
- **Quality of life and adaptation**: knowledge, skills and collaborative participation.
- **Social and cultural influences**: health beliefs, professional cultural competence, access to and appropriateness of services and social perceptions of disability.
- **Financial impacts**: availability of income and insurance and the demand for specific needs-led resources.
- **Professional interventions**: attitudes, knowledge and skills, resource allocation and legislation.

Such information will require a depth of assessment that is beyond the scope of the two PARR predictive models and most likely beyond the resources of most community-based healthcare workers. Such depth of assessment will demand data drawn from the continuum of health and social care support and be gathered over a period of time. In order to collect and collate such information, the Department of Health through the consortium of the King's Fund, New York University and Health Dialog have developed the combined predictive model. This model links primary and secondary care events to provide risk stratification related to the likelihood of future high-frequency use of secondary care services. It does not rely on prior hospital admission as the trigger and is therefore potentially more of an asset to case finding, being pre-emptive in organising care services to reduce the interruption of lifestyle and cost of hospital admission.

The combined (predictive) model uses risk stratification at four levels offering the opportunity to assess those who will hold the greatest risk of emergency admission (see Figure 3.2).

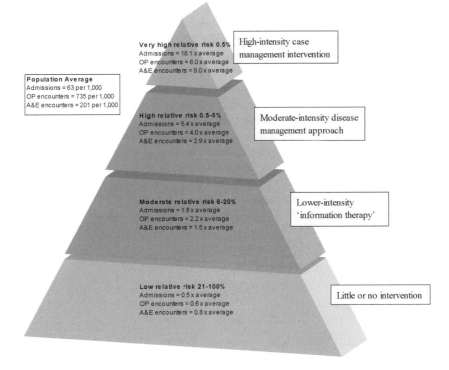

Very high relative risk 0.5%
Admissions = 18.1 x average
OP encounters = 6.0 x average
A&E encounters = 9.0 x average

High-intensity case management intervention

Population Average
Admissions = 63 per 1,000
OP encounters = 735 per 1,000
A&E encounters = 201 per 1,000

High relative risk 0.5-5%
Admissions = 5.4 x average
OP encounters = 4.0 x average
A&E encounters = 2.9 x average

Moderate-intensity disease management approach

Moderate relative risk 6-20%
Admissions = 1.8 x average
OP encounters = 2.2 x average
A&E encounters = 1.5 x average

Lower-intensity 'information therapy'

Low relative risk 21-100%
Admissions = 0.5 x average
OP encounters = 0.6 x average
A&E encounters = 0.8 x average

Little or no intervention

Figure 3.2 Risk stratification of population
Source: King's Fund et al., 2006a

This stratification identifies 0.5% of the population hold 18.6 more chance of hospital admission than the average person and as such are most likely to require case management and outreach targeted interventions. It is argued that as well as identifying those at such high risk, the model will equally predict those at the lower end of risk stratification, thereby facilitating the development of health promotion activities in the low-risk group, specific supported care for those at moderate risk and early and timely intervention for those at high and very high risk. From a fiscal perspective it is expected effective intervention would reduce the impact of illness by 20%, with corresponding financial savings, (King's Fund et al., 2006a).

The combined model considered more than 850 variables including values drawn from administrative records, social services (this was later withdrawn from the study due to an inability to match data), general practice, accident and emergency and inpatient encounters and from pharmaceutical support and pathological investigations. Each was subject to time periods to account for the occurrence and patterns of recurrence. Clinical profiles included asthma, COPD, depression, diabetes, hypertension, cancer and coronary heart disease/heart failure, with further specialist codes (ICD-10) identifying a much greater number of diagnoses. Data was extrapolated from medication prescriptions, e.g. the presence of prescribed hypertensive medication was taken to indicate a hypertensive illness. More data was drawn from the number of medications prescribed or taken, average age and gender and the average length of stay following emergency admission (King's Fund et al., 2006a). Patients were identified through NHS number or through the patient administration system (PAS) number.

The preceding sections are an impossibly shortened version of the methodology and is provided not to inform further technical studies but to offer a clinical perception of the scope of the database. Applied locally, this predictive model could offer a well-informed stratification of the population's needs that could then be segmented to formulate a caseload. The model does require access to a minimum of two years' historical data, which in itself may not be totally reliable across a primary care trust (PCT). In order to facilitate this, the work of PARR 1 and PARR 2 would provide a baseline from which to proceed.

Data storage

The data collected will require systematic storage. In predictive modelling terms, this is 'warehousing'. The 'warehouse' is a common repository that offers information about patients from different sources. In the King's Fund study these sources were acute service involvement, outpatient involvement, accident and emergency use and general practice attendance. An inclusion criterion was set to be any person who had an encounter with health services in the past two years. An example of the quantitative findings for two PCTs taken from the King's Fund study is given in Table 3.1.

Table 3.1 Warehouse representation

	Records	
	PCT 1	*PCT 4*
Inpatient	151,546	111,999
Outpatient	1,223,546	323,568
A&E	195,582	70,406
General practice	14,926,771	5,829,098

Source: Kings Fund et al., 2006a: 53

From these figures the broad numbers of people using the services may be recognised but there is now a need to identify potential patients.

As seen, the combined predictive tool sets variables for prediction within the sources of data: inpatient (IP), outpatient (OP), A&E and general practice (GP) (see Box 3.1). Through accessing the NHS/PAS number it is possible to identify those people who make up the statistics – to develop the membership list – and, through comparing frequency of use, segment the population at different levels of need.

Box 3.1 Sources of data and predictors (combined predictive tool)

IP data:

- disease conditions
- utilisation (types of admission)
- ICD codes with multiple use where multiple conditions exist
- number of day cases

OP data:

- number of OP visits
- number of medical specialist visits
- attendance record, onward referrals

A&E data:

- number of A&E visits
- length of stay, arrival mode, sub-categorization of site on body

GP data:

- appliances and equipment
- cause of injury
- clinical findings
- medications, including poly-pharmacy
- operations and procedures
- routine laboratory results plus HbA1c, cholesterol, GFR and FEV
- lifestyle including smoking status, BP, alcohol consumption and BMI

Alternatively, work between Imperial College London and University College, London, has resulted in the high-impact user manager (HUM) system. This system uses hospital episodes statistics (HES) to predict future admissions through identifying specific conditions brought under the umbrella term of ambulatory care-sensitive conditions (ACSs). A list of ACSs is provided on the HUM webpage (Drfosterintelligence, 2007), but in essence they are conditions that are responsive to timely intervention to reduce hospital admissions.

The HUM sets definitions for high- and very high-impact users, basically under the threshold approach, with high-impact users being people who have undertaken at least three emergency admissions within a 12-month period and have at least one ACS condition. Very high-impact users will have undertaken at least nine admissions in the past three years, with at least one in each of the three calendar years. In the latter, diagnosis has no bearing. However, this system upgrades from the threshold approach through adopting *regression modelling* to determine the relationship between the ACS conditions and other variables. Demographic, quality of life, social and cultural variables have been included in a regression statistical analysis offering an improved predictive value for a limited range of conditions. This aspect has increased the popularity of the model among community matrons, although the limitations of data being three months old and the fact of the model being acute admission dependent are noted.

Summary

In summary, the data does exist for case finding but the processes involved are not well aligned. Such data is complex and cross-agency and even cross-practice data is often incompatible for analysis. The accumulation and dissemination of useful data at trust level does not have a high priority, resulting in poor information routes creating huge time gaps. In practice, case finding is following the disease management model. These factors make case finding more response driven than proactive, despite the demand to predict and reduce future service use. Current prediction models are fast developing and it is foreseeable that such models will soon outstrip current IT capability across agencies, bringing some frustration to implementing predictive case finding. Meanwhile, current systems of care do not offer a clear context in which to define case finding. It is arguable that case finding should engage a wide range of needs in order to develop proactivity, but the demand to prove short-term benefit in terms of avoiding hospital admission will by its nature focus on high-intensity users. It is hoped this chapter will provoke reflection on case finding as an aspect of case management and in terms of recognising the capacity of practitioners working in the role.

It is clear from the literature that case finding is an organisational challenge and not merely the role of the advanced practitioner. The benefits are predicted in terms of user quality of life and in financial return for providers and yet there is little focus from providers at this time. National efforts have produced a number of approaches that need to be understood and used appropriately. Predictive modelling cannot be the sole domain of administrators but requires additional knowledge and skills found in clinicians. Within the approach, the practitioner should be wary of single-strand development. Individuals and communities are complex and require a number of strategies to arrive at practical and beneficial outcomes.

At its basis, case finding must be successful in meeting the needs of the individual user. The model must fit the user and not have the user shaped to fit the model. Lubkin and Larsen's 'predictive features' may be key in applying a population risk strategy. There does need to be local clarity around the process of case finding and within this the identification of people with the right skills and knowledge to meet local needs. The concept of case finding being the domain of the practitioner must be explored and expanded within the local provider organisation.

References

Department of Health (DH) (2005) *National Service Framework for Long-Term (Neurological) Conditions*. London, DH.

King's Fund, Health Dialog Analytic Solutions, New York University (2006a) *Combined Predictive Model, Final Report*. http://www.kingsfund.org.uk/applications/forms/combinedmodel_download.rm (accessed 03/08/07).

King's Fund, Health Dialog Analytic Solutions, New York University (2006b) *Case-finding Algorithms for Patients at Risk of Re-Hospitalisation. PARR 1 and PARR 2*. http://www.kingsfund.org.uk/current_projects/predictive_risk/patients_at_risk.html (accessed 03/08/07).

Lubkin, I. and Larsen, P. (2002) *Chronic Illness Impact and Interventions*. London, Jones & Bartlett.

McCain, J. (2001) *Predictive Modelling holds Promise of Earlier Identification and Treatment*. www.managedcaremag.com/archives/0109/0109.predictive.html (accessed 27/07/07).

NHS Modernisation Agency and Skills for Health (2005a) *Case Management Competence Framework for the Care of People with Long-term Conditions*. London, NHS Modernisation Agency and Skills for Health.

NHS Modernisation Agency and Skills for Health (2005b) *Predictive Risk Project. Best practice guidance*. London, NHS Modernisation Agency and Skills for Health.

Ozer, K. and Cilingiroglu, M. (2007) *Vulnerable Plaque: definition, detection, treatment and future implications, Current Medicine Group LLC*. www.springerlink.com (accessed 27/07/07).

Patel, U., Murdoch, I. and Theodossiades, J. (2006) Glaucoma detection in the community. *Eye* 20, 5, 591–594.

Porter, B., Macfarlane, R., Unwin, N. and Walker, R. (2006) The prevalence of Parkinson's disease in an area of North Tyneside in the Northeast of England. *Neuroepidemiology* 26, 3, 156–161.

Sanders, D., Patel, D., Khan, F., Westbrook, R., Webber, C., Milford-Ward, A. et al. (2005) Case finding for adults celiac disease in patients with reduced bone mineral density. *Digestive Disease and Sciences* 50, 3, 587–592.

University of Birmingham (2006) *Improving Care for People with Long Term Conditions – a review of UK and international frameworks*. London, HMSO.

Vandevoorde, J., Verbanck, S., Gijssels, L., Schuermans, D., Devroey, D., DeBacker, J. et al. (2007) Early detection of COPD: a case finding study in general practice. *Respiratory Medicine* 101, 3, 525–530.

www.drfosterintelligence.co.uk/managementInformation/HUM (accessed 13/08/07).

4 Case management

Sarah Lewis

Introduction

The context of care is changing; we now have an ageing population and an increase in chronic illnesses (DH, 1999, 2005a; WHO, 2002) that will demand more complex and costly care over a longer timeframe. With the NHS facing increased pressure on acute hospital beds and finances, the importance of maintaining people in their own homes or community has become increasingly pertinent.

A public service agreement target was announced by the Department of Health in 2004 calling for a reduction in emergency bed days by 5% by 2008 (DH, 2004a). This is set against the known trend of continual increases in emergency admissions, many of which are for patients with chronic diseases (Hutt et al., 2004). A chronic disease is defined as a condition that requires ongoing medical care that can only control not cure, limits what one can do and is likely to last longer than one year (DH, 2004b; NHS Modernisation Agency, 2005) (See Table 4.1).

Table 4.1 Impact of chronic disease

Global issue	National issue
Healthcare challenge of the century	17.5 million people in this country report a long-term condition
Leading cause of disability by 2020	Up to 80% of GP consultations are connected to chronic conditions
If not managed effectively will become the most expensive problem facing healthcare	60% of hospital bed days are for patients with chronic disease

Source: Global issue: WHO 2002; DH 2004b, 2005b; National issue: NHS Modernisation Agency 2005; DH 2004b, 2005b

The management of chronic disease became a national priority and frameworks were detailed in the NHS Plan (DH, 2000), the NHS Improvement Plan (DH, 2004c) and subsequent policy documents specifically related to the management of long-term conditions. Current policy recognises the need for effective management of long-term conditions, achieved in part by liberating the talents of nurses in primary care (DH, 2002, 2005c) and a move away from an acute, episodic model of care focused on urgent need to a proactive one (DH, 2000; WHO 2002). The introduction of national service frameworks and the new GMS contract further added to the drive for case management of chronic disease (Young, 2005).

Background

The term case management originated in North America in the 1950s to describe the care given to community psychiatric patients (Lee et al., 1998). At the start of the 1980s it developed into a strategy running alongside managed care to contain the costs of and focus the care of older people. It came to the forefront in the 1990s when Medicaid, a healthcare scheme for older people, was revised to include the increasing provision of home and community care (Kane, 2000).

In the United Kingdom, case management is a term used to describe a range of strategies that improve the coordination of services for people with complex needs. There is no one single model but a range of approaches that plan, coordinate, manage and review the care of an individual (Hutt et al., 2004). Case management involves working proactively with primary health-care teams and patients to draw up personal plans for those who are identified as high-intensity service users or are at risk of hospital admissions. The aim is to improve quality of life and coordinate care in the context of efficiency and cost effectiveness.

Some forms of case management have existed in the NHS for the last two decades in areas such as social care, mental health and specialist services and it is often referred to as care management, with the two terms used inter-changeably. Case management formed the centrepiece of the NHS and Community Care Act 1991, where it was called care management. Today it is a concept used to address the increasing challenge of long-term illness conditions.

The government's strategy for long-term conditions encompasses three population management approaches to care: case management, disease management and support for self-management (Hutt et al., 2004):

- **Case management** is aimed at the limited group of patients (around 3% to 5% of the population) who have two or more long-term conditions with health and social care needs that become dis-proportionately more complex (DH, 2004b).
- **Disease management**, the next step down, is aimed at patients with one long-term condition. Through the use of clinical pathways

and protocols they are managed with support from a multi-disciplinary team on a disease-oriented basis (DH, 2004b).

- **Self-management**, the final layer, covers the majority of the population who are supported to take an active role in managing their own condition (DH, 2004b) with support from healthcare professionals and initiatives such as the expert patient programme.

Case management is not confined to one professional group and elements of it should be incorporated into all healthcare professionals' roles to ensure the concept is all-encompassing along the patient's journey. The diversity of approaches and varied interventions allows for this as it is aimed at a diverse population across various settings (Hutt et al., 2004). All the case management models proclaim significant roles for nurses because of their broad assessment and coordination skills and contain an emphasis on the management of long-term conditions.

Core elements of case management

Wherever case management is applied and in whatever setting it is used, it should consist of six core elements:

- case finding or screening
- assessment
- care planning
- coordination and referral/implementation
- monitoring
- review (Hutt et al., 2004).

This approach is similar to the nursing process, the features that distinguish case management involving the above elements from similar approaches (Hutt et al., 2004) such as facilitated discharge and intermediate care are:

- intensity of involvement
- breadth of services spanned
- duration of involvement.

Identifying the population at risk

Before case management can commence, potential patients need to be identified. By stratifying the patient population to identify those at risk of unplanned hospital admissions and providing more secondary care in the community (DH, 2002) will go toward meeting the public service agreement targets (DH, 2005d). Often by case finding, patients are identified that have low levels or no input from health or social care services in the way of preventive or ongoing care. These patients can be allocated a case manager and given support on a proactive basis to improve their health and allow them to remain independent for as long as possible.

To identify the target population for case management, criteria need to be applied and these vary between the model of case management adopted but include some of the following principles:

- 65 years old or over (some are over 18 years)
- two or more active long-term conditions
- two or more unplanned admissions to hospital in the last 12 months
- two or more GP visits in past three months
- identified at risk by clinical judgment
- four or more prescribed medications.

(See Chapter 3 for more information about case finding.)

Assessment and care planning

Comprehensive needs assessment in collaboration with the patient and their family identifies unmet needs and current functional ability. Exacerbations of long-term illness conditions can be identified earlier on and treated on a timely basis to prevent unnecessary hospital admissions. This will be an ongoing process and include the expertise of other practitioners within the multiagency team as required. The assessment must be recorded along with future planning, including wishes and shared with all involved in the patients care (Rossi, 1999). This will need to include out-of-hours services and other relevant parties such as the ambulance service and the local acute NHS trust. In addition the Darzi review of the NHS (DH, 2008) states that all patients with a long term condition should have an individualised care plan by 2010.

Coordination/referral/implementation

Integrating all elements of care and being a single point of contact for the patient and their family is a requirement and strength of case management. Communicating the plan of care to all other healthcare professionals involved is vital such as the GP, district nurse and secondary care staff such as consultants and staff on the wards during any admissions. This can lead to integrated working and swift facilitated discharges as the patient's normal level of functioning and level of support will be known by the case manager.

Monitoring

Promoting self-management and the expert patient model, such as in diabetes care where education can improve understanding and control of the condition, can be beneficial to the patient. Any changes in health can be identified quickly and the right treatment arranged at the right time to avoid crisis situations.

Review

Patients and their families can plan for the future to make the most appropriate choices for them over their health and have those decisions open for discussion. Opportunities to change medications, care packages or end-of-life plans may arise and can then be shared with the multiagency team to ensure the patient's wishes are upheld.

Models of case management

Of the different models of case management no one model has been found to be superior to the others. Each PCT should configure a model suitable to the needs of its target population (Hutt et al., 2004) and choose and adapt the models accordingly. There are four main models of case management: Evercare, Kaiser, Pfizer and Unique Care; they differ in their approaches, implementation and focus (see *Table 4.2.*)

Evercare model of case management

Evercare was founded by two nurse practitioners in 1987 in Minnesota who wanted to reduce fragmentation in the care of older people, the disabled and the chronically ill. Evercare is part of a division of UnitedHealth Group dedicated to older people's needs. It sought to foster ongoing relationships with patients and all those involved in their care across community, primary and secondary care (Evercare, 2007). Evercare has become the United States of America's largest programme for older people, recognised for its innovation in health and managing health care costs (Evercare, 2007). The scheme successfully moved away from episodic care and employed nurse practitioners to coordinate a proactive approach starting with the identification of those at highest risk of unplanned hospital admissions (UnitedHealth Europe, 2005).

In the UK nine PCTs piloted the Evercare model with direct input from the UnitedHealth Group to see if similar benefits could be produced within the NHS (UnitedHealth Europe, 2005). A project team was set up and a high-risk population enrolled in the programme. A high-risk individual was

Table 4.2 The four main models of case management

	Evercare	**Kaiser**	**Pfizer**	**Unique**
Overall aim	Case management targeted at those with highest risk of hospital admission	Management of disease by population Focus on integrated services	Case management targeted at those at highest risk by disease severity	Case management targeted at those at highest risk by disease severity/risk of hospital admissions
Lead practitioner	Advanced primary nurses Competency-based guidelines for advanced practice	Clinical leaders across primary and secondary care	Care managers and nurses Informacare© decision support software	District nurses Social workers
Approach	Individualized/ holistic Interdisciplinary Multidisciplinary care plan Medicines management	Group consultation Integrated care pathways Discharge planners Patient education on website and during hospital admissions	Coaching over the telephone Encourage self-management Assessment and management Local and national guidelines	Practice-based management Individualized/ holistic care plans Multidisciplinary Medicines management
Partnership working	Advanced-level nurse General practitioner Consultant Spans primary and secondary care	Clinicians Managers	Acute trusts Local stakeholders	General practitioner Practice team Social worker Acute trust Spans primary and secondary care

identified as someone over 65 years of age, with two or more unplanned hospital admissions within the last 12 months. At the time this was the only data-driven method available.

The Evercare model has five key principles:

- **Individualized approach** where the team gets to know the patient and other healthcare professionals involved in their care, resulting in personalised care that aids communication. Ninety-five percent of patients involved in the UK project saw an improvement in their ability to cope and felt fully involved in their care (UnitedHealth Europe, 2005).
- **Centred on primary care** where care is integrated through medical, health and social needs with nurse practitioners or social

workers taking the lead (Evercare, 2007). The Evercare pilot evaluation in the UK saw a fall in the number of GP home visits for the top two groups at highest risk of unplanned admissions (Boaden et al., 2006). This was due in part to proactive visits by nurse practitioners, who were able to identify problems early and teach patients how to recognise and respond to exacerbations of their long-term illness condition.

- **Proactive, systematic approach** with care in the least invasive manner in the least invasive setting. The UK study demonstrated a reduction in unplanned hospital admissions by 38%. Of those in the GP-nominated group who had not had any unplanned admissions, the rate increased from 21 to 62 (UnitedHealth Europe, 2005). This increase could be explained as inevitable; they were identified as high risk for admission so there should be no surprise that this happened. Equally, regression towards the mean for the high-admissions group could explain the fall in admissions (UnitedHealth Europe, 2005) from a statistical point of view.
- **Medicines management** incorporating medication reviews. The UK pilot highlighted that, while there was no overall reduction in medications taken, some potentially harmful medications were reduced or alternatives given (Rossi, 1999; UnitedHealth Europe, 2005).
- **Data-rich approach**, to identify vulnerable patients, measure performance, evaluate and benchmark care (Evercare, 2003). The pilot site only had access to emergency admission data to case find, whereas the programme in the USA uses this alongside data on clinical conditions, medications and other health and social care input to case find (UnitedHealth Europe, 2005).

The Evercare pilot was only in place for eight months (UnitedHealth Europe, 2005), which is far too early in the implementation of the programme to expect significant results. The nurse practitioners in the pilot would not have had time to develop all the skills needed; for example, many prescribing courses take over six months to complete. This also allowed no time for organisational changes such as an increase in care managers or access to respite beds to support the service. There is great potential in this role and it needs to be allowed to develop fully and be supported by all involved to make it a success.

Kaiser Permanente's model of case management

Kaiser's approach to case management is similar to that of Evercare and can be compared to the NHS, as the per capita costs of the two systems, allowing for adjustments in benefits and the cost environment, were similar to within 10% of each other (Feachem et al., 2002). Kaiser costs about the same to run as the NHS but performs considerably better in areas such as prompt diagnosis and treatment. Kaiser provides a similar range of services and have had the same time to evolve as an organisation making them comparable (Feachem et al., 2002).

Primary care physicians working within the Kaiser principles can perform complex procedures in their clinics freeing up the time of specialists and consultants in secondary care. The roles of physicians assistants and nurse practitioners have been developed and they can diagnose, prescribe and case manage patients, increasing the numbers of case managers overall (Feachem et al., 2002; Matrix Research and Consultancy, 2004). The approach in the UK is similar but on a smaller scale with community matrons able to diagnose, prescribe and manage caseloads. This goes some way to explain why Kaiser has signifcantly lower bed day use, as it monitors admissions closely, reduces length of stay, has many chronic disease management programmes and offers physician appointments in the evening and weekends to avoid emergency department visits (Feachem et al., 2002).

In the USA, Kaiser has achieved real integration through all components of the healthcare system (Feachem et al., 2002; Singh, 2005) avoiding payments to other providers of care and allowing the patient to be cared for in the most appropriate setting without penalty. Integration in the NHS is somewhat fragmented with some PCTs having already integrated health and social care successfully and others only just considering such integration.

Pfizer's model of case management

Pfizer Ltd, a UK-based pharmaceutical company, launched a 15-month pilot in 2004 providing individualised support for patients in a London borough. Six hundred patients with coronary heart disease, heart failure and/or diabetes were case managed by four case managers who provided individualised support and arranged interventions with the aid of Pfizer Health Solutions InformaCare decision support software. As with other models the patients were identified as being high risk by disease severity, outpatient and secondary care usage (Chamberlain-Webber, 2004). This approach was carried out using telephone care management with the nurses coaching the patients in good management and signposting services they may benefit from. While this approach focuses on those at highest risk of hospital admission, it relies on the recruitment of care managers to provide telephone support rather than a 'hands-on' clinical approach. This fosters great coordination of care but on a limited basis as some aspects of care such as medication reviews or complex assessments are not included as dedicated elements of this approach (Matrix Research and Consultancy, 2004).

Unique model of case management

The Castlefields model, also known as the Unique model was set up in a group practice in Runcorn that serves 12,000 patients. The approach has reduced emergency hospital admissions by 15% (DH, 2004b). Although based on active management of long-term conditions it pulled on elements of case management with good success, targeting those who have had unplanned hospital admissions and those with health and social care needs (DH, 2005c). A nurse case manages each patient and works closely with social services meaning more timely and appropriate referrals. This approach works well enabling patients to be case managed as staff have dedicated time for the role; how well this would work if applied across a population remains to be seen.

Effectiveness of case management

The effectiveness of case management has been brought into question with many people citing weak evidence of its ability to reduce hospital admissions (Hutt et al., 2004; Gravelle et al., 2007). One of the main aspects of case management reported as evidence was the impact on emergency admission rates. These have been inconsistent and fluctuating and will need to be studied over a longer timeframe to monitor the progress of admissions for patients who are case managed. Similarly, length of stay has been shown in some studies to have decreased for case-managed patients (Hutt et al., 2004); however, some studies show no significant effects (Gravelle et al., 2007). *Case study 4.1* highlights these issues and achievements in practice.

Case study 4.1 Patient managed by a community matron (CM) based on Evercare model

Rita is an 81-year-old lady who lives alone in her own home within a rural community. She is a widow and has no children. The CM highlighted her high number of admissions from admissions data from the local acute trust.

On assessment the following was found:

- **PMH**: COPD, type 1 diabetes, osteoarthritis and a recent CVA leaving her with a mild residual weakness on one side and poor short-term memory. On discharge, she had a care package of one call a day in the morning to assist with personal hygiene.
- She had three admissions in the previous six months for exacerbations of her COPD and diabetes.

Case management over the next year included:

- Weekly support visits from the CM.
- Very high-intensity service user (VHISU) assessment document kept in the patient's home, updated every three months and sent to her GP/out of hours services/ambulance trust.
- Monthly GP VHISU meetings to discuss case and plan care with multi-disciplinary team.
- Six-monthly medication reviews and nurse prescribing by CM.
- Patient and carer education and support with medication/lifestyle/diet/COPD/diabetes/osteoarthritis.
- Ongoing liaison with GP/specialist nurses/social workers.
- Carers increased to three calls a day to assist with meals and shopping.
- Two exacerbations of COPD managed at home as detected early, diabetes well controlled.

Admissions for the following year while under case management:

- One admission for a transient ischaemic attack (TIA).
- Early discharge facilitated by attending ward rounds, liaising with ward staff and a good knowledge of her previous capabilities, care provision and home set-up.

Weak evidence has been cited as causative of these findings; however, Hutt et al. (2004) recognise that the evidence is neither positive nor conclusive. Case management is a relatively new concept for the management of long-term conditions management and new roles are still very much developmental. Some studies recognise that these roles are unlikely to produce results until there is more radical system design with full establishment and integration (Gravelle et al. 2007). Case management needs to be fully evaluated here in the UK but it needs to be given time to develop and for the infrastructure to support new ways of working. The government set a target of 3000 community matrons in post by 2008; many, if not all, will need to develop the skills required, so will not be able to take on the role in its entirety for some time. Three thousand community matrons across the whole of England and Wales is a relatively small number, so significant results cannot be expected until these numbers increase and those in post attain the full potential of their role.

Skills for effective case management

The NHS Modernisation Agency (2005) has developed a set of competencies for case management across nine domains with over 100 competencies in all. They have been designed to help practitioners working in case management to implement the National Service Framework for Long-term Conditions (DH, 2005b). They will ensure common standards across the country and their competency base provides a guiding framework to define the role, keeping it clinical and in accordance with Agenda for Change's knowledge and skills focus.

Community matrons and those working as case managers need to demonstrate competence in all domains; however, an emphasis on advanced clinical nursing practice is specific to the community matron role. This domain closely follows the requirements for advanced practitioners set by the Nursing and Midwifery Council (NMC). As the role involves providing clinical care at an advanced level, competence will need to be demonstrated through master's level practice (NHS Modernisation Agency, 2005). Case managers who work autonomously will need to acquire some or all of the remaining competencies also at master's level. In their review of case management, Hutt et al. (2004) found that most community matrons were nurses, but not exclusively, they often had master's level qualifications or were studying towards them. They had extensive experience with older people or in chronic disease management and were required to develop skills, such as self-directed learning, managing risk, authority to act on behalf of patients, higher level communication and negotiation skills.

Advanced clinical nursing practice

The community matron role is highly autonomous and will involve history taking, advanced assessment, physical examination, diagnosis and prescribing and having access to intermediate care and referral rights to consultants. This requires the individual practitioner to be accountable for their practice at this level with much of the role undertaken alone, with minimal supervision.

Supervision (Hutt et al., 2004) and mentorship is vital if advanced practice is to be fostered; however, one of the biggest challenges is finding suitably qualified mentors. So far many advanced practitioners have looked to the medical profession to provide mentorship, as highlighted by the Evercare project in the UK (UnitedHealth Europe, 2005). To date, mentorship has been fragmented but as current community matrons and advanced practitioners develop they can mentor future practitioners (see Chapter 8 for more information on mentorship).

Leading complex care coordination

Systems need to be in place to support this, such as information technology (IT) facilities that allow all health professional to access the patients' jointly-held IT records rather than each professional having their own record that is unavailable to others. Training in these systems, concept and practical application of case management (Hutt et al., 2004) is vital for it to be understood and applied by all to foster collaborative working.

Proactively manage long-term conditions

Strong clinical and leadership skills will be vital to act as the coordinator and lead care, rather than being subservient to the orders of the medical profession. A sound knowledge of resources is vital to access equipment and services for patents on a timely basis.

Managing cognitive impairment and mental well-being

Mental health conditions such as dementia and Alzheimer's disease are long-term conditions that require effective management. Understanding the condition, its manifestations, decline and the strain it places on the person and their family are vital for effective care. Organising support for families or carers in the form of information, respite, voluntary agencies, carers to assist with social needs and day centre care can be beneficial. These measures can prevent carer fatigue and enable the patient to remain in their own home if appropriate and remain flexible to adapt to changing or increasing needs.

Supporting self-care, self-management and enabling independence

Skills to empower patients and enable them to self-care are invaluable, such as providing alternative devises for self-administering insulin that can be used with people who have reduced dexterity.

Professional practice and leadership

Engaging commissioners fully to ensure that the pathway for case management and the community matron role can be fully developed and integrated into the system is imperative. Providing evidence for the role to date through outcomes and case studies will be invaluable here to prove the worth of the approach. This is vital if the role of community matrons are understood by all key players (DH, 2005c). Indeed, this is a poignant lesson learnt in the experience of many nurse consultants.

Identifying high-risk patients, promoting health and preventing ill health

Developing better ways to identify high-risk patients that incorporate all their data not just admissions details will add to the role and ensure the right patients are targeted (see Chapter 3 for further information on case finding).

Managing care at the end of life

Having a sound knowledge of the disease process to allow the assessment of the advanced and terminal stages of life allows the patient and family to prepare and plan for dying. Their wishes can be shared with the family and planning for the terminal phase undertaken.

Interagency and partnership working

Often many patients have a complex mix of health and social care needs and require coordination of services around those needs. Their case manager will coordinate all these services, review them regularly and act as a single point of contact to everyone including the patients. Developing close links between primary and secondary care is useful. This is aided by case managers following patients into secondary care at admission to aid discharge and to share the patient's wishes with staff in the acute setting. Setting up regular meetings with those involved with case managing patients to discuss care, share ideas about options and good practice and ensure everyone is updated on each patient and new initiatives is particularly useful.

Summary

Current government policy indicates that case management is here to stay; however, the wider disease agenda must not be forgotten. The majority of patients with a single long-term condition today have the potential to become the complex cases of tomorrow, unless the chronic disease agenda pushes forward as a whole.

The challenges ahead include engaging staff in the case management approach, enabling the change process and overcoming resistance to achieve the outcomes of the approach. Rapid access to good-quality data and support for the development of the case manager and community matron role could see a significant impact on the lives of patients with complex long-term conditions.

References

Boaden, R., Dusheiko, M., Gravelle, H. Parker, S., Pickard, S., Roland, M. et al. (2006) *Evercare Evaluation: final report*. Manchester, National Primary Care Research and Development Centre.

Chamberlain-Webber, J. (2004) Tackling chronic disease. *Professional Nurse* 20, 4, 14–18.

Department of Health (DH) (1999) *Making a Difference: strengthening the nursing, midwifery and health visiting contribution to health and healthcare*. London, HMSO.

Department of Health (DH) (2000) *The NHS Plan: a plan for investment, a plan for reform*. London, HMSO.

Department of Health (DH) (2002) *Liberating the Talents*. London, HMSO.

Department of Health (DH) (2004a) *Improving Chronic Disease Management*. London, DH.

Department of Health (DH) (2004b) *Chronic Disease Management: a compendium of information*. London, DH.

Department of Health (DH) (2004c) *The NHS Improvement Plan: putting people at the heart of public services*. London, DH.

Department of Health (DH) (2005a) *Supporting People with Long-term Conditions*. London, DH.

Department of Health (DH) (2005b) *The National Service Framework for Long-term Conditions*. London, DH.

Department of Health (DH) (2005c) *Supporting People with Long-term Conditions: liberating the talents of nurses who care for people with long-term conditions*. London, DH.

Department of Health (DH) (2005d) *Supporting People with Long-Term Conditions: an NHS and social care model to support local innovation and integration*. London, DH.

Department of Health (2008) *NHS Next Stage Review. Our vision for Primary and Community Care*. London, DH.

Evercare (2007) *Newsroom*. http://www.evercarehealthplans.com/newsroom_article3.jsp (accessed 08/05/2007).

Feachem, R., Sekhri, N. and White, K. (2002) Getting more for their dollar: a comparison of the NHS with California's Kaiser Permanente. *British Medical Journal* 324, 135–143.

Gravelle, H., Dusheiko, M., Sheaff, R., Sargent, P. Boaden, R., Pickard, S. et al. (2007) Impact of case management (Evercare) on frail elderly patients: controlled before and after analysis of quantitative outcome data. *British Medical Journal* 334, 7583, 31–34.

Hutt, R., Rosen, R. and McCauley, J. (2004) *Case Managing Long-term Conditions: what impact does it have in the treatment of older people?* London, King's Fund.

Kane, S. (2000) The implementation of the Evercare demonstration project. *Journal of the American Geriatric Society* 48, 2, 218–223.

Lee, D., Mackenzie, A., Dudley-Brown, S. and Chin, T. (1998) Case management: a review of the definitions and practices. *Journal of Advanced Nursing* 27, 5, 933–939.

Matrix Research and Consultancy (2004) *Learning Distillation of Chronic Disease Management Programmes in the UK*. London, DH.

NHS Modernisation Agency (2005) *Case Management Competencies Framework*. London, DH.

Rossi, P. (1999) *Case Management in Healthcare: a practical guide*. Philadelphia, PA, W.B. Saunders Company.

Singh, D. (2005) *Transforming Chronic Care: evidence about improving care for people with long-term conditions*. Birmingham, University of Birmingham and Surrey and Sussex PCT Alliance.

UnitedHealth Europe (2005) *Assessment of the Evercare Programme in England 2003–2004*. London, UnitedHealth Group Company.

World Health Organisation (WHO) (2002) *Innovative Care for Chronic Conditions: Building Blocks for Action*. Geneva, WHO.

Young, L. (2005) Supporting people with long-term conditions. *Primary Health Care* 15, 2, 12–13.

5 First contact and complex needs assessment

Lucy Botting

Introduction

Over the last 20 years traditional nursing boundaries have become increasingly blurred. Twenty years ago nurses were conditioned to a nursing assessment based around the gathering of information of a patient's physiological, psychological, sociological and spiritual needs encompassed within a holistic assessment framework, dictated by the style of the appropriate nursing model, for example, Roper, Logan and Tierney or Orem (Aggleton and Chalmers, 2000). The purpose of this stage was to identify the patients' 'nursing' problems and hence develop a plan suitable to meet patients' needs.

In 2004 the Royal College of Nursing (RCN) stated that an assessment should be the first step towards the process of individualised nursing care, providing information critical towards the development of an action plan enhancing personal health status. The RCN also suggested this plan should decrease the potential for, or severity of, chronic long-term conditions (RCN, 2004).

While these statements may be true to those studying at pre-registration level, emphasis within post-registration education has moved on in tandem with the changing climate of healthcare in relation to both political and governmental influences and based around the demographic societal trends within the United Kingdom. For instance, at the time of writing, higher education institutions (HEIs) are very much open to debate about the course content of the district nursing post-registration programme. Some universities have now decided to amalgamate elements of the advanced practitioner–community matron modules within the programme, while others watch and wait.

Twenty-first-century complex needs assessment: a differential diagnosis

Post-registration education and training within the primary care setting does not prepare the nurse for the demands of dealing with the complexities of assessment at an advanced level. Patients with undifferentiated diagnosis and complex problems demand that the health professional practises with a higher degree of autonomy and has advanced level skills and knowledge. As a consequence physical assessment and diagnostic skills need to be learnt allied with thorough history taking and clinical decision-making skills. The concept of nurses undertaking a consultation is relatively new and theoretical models such as Byrne and Long (1976), Stott and Davies (1979), Pendleton et al. (1984) and the Calgary–Cambridge model (Silverman et al., 1998) may prove useful as a guiding framework.

Traditionally diagnosis has been seen as the prerogative of the medical practitioner with nurses' involvement being informal and often unacknowledged (Baird, 2001). In reaching a working diagnosis the practitioner will go through several stages of data collection and analysis. Bates (1995) discusses in some depth the process of clinical decision making and establishing a working diagnosis while acknowledging that it is not always possible to reach such a definitive diagnosis.

The following section will go some way to exploring a guiding framework through which the practitioner may be able to ascertain such a working diagnosis.

History taking

Taking a history prior to physical examination allows the practitioner an insight into important information about the patient's health needs. It is the most important primary skill in the assessment process and is the key to a correct clinical diagnosis. In a sense the interview or consultation should be viewed as the meeting of two experts: the patient, an expert on the experience of his/her illness, and the clinician, an expert on diagnosis and management of illness.

For new patients in hospital or within a long-term care setting the practitioner will need to complete a comprehensive health history. For patients who seek care for a specific complaint such as painful urination or a chest infection, i.e. for those within a walk-in-centre environment, a more limited interview tailored to the specific problem is indicated. Bates (2007) calls this a focused or problem-oriented history.

History-taking techniques

Eliciting accurate detailed and unbiased information from a patient is a skilled task and not simply a matter of recording the patient's responses to a series of questions. A study by Ramsey et al. (1998) concluded that even physicians miss important patient information during their initial consultation and advocated the use of a checklist to ensure a full history was elicited and hence diagnosis and treatment was accurate (see *Box 5.1*).

Box 5.1 Top 10 techniques to eliciting a history

1. The practitioner should give patients an environment conducive to producing a thorough history and give the patient their undivided attention.
2. Medical records should be reviewed before the consultation and note taking kept to a minimum when the patient is talking.
3. The patient must be able to understand the language utilised by the practitioner. Use of translation technology may aid this process.
4. The practitioner should not interrupt the patient and should allow the patient to tell their story in their own words.
5. Patients should be steered towards relevant details.
6. Open questions should be used initially with specific (closed questions) thereafter.
7. The practitioner should clarify any lay terms or words a patient uses to describe illness.
8. History should include events up to the day of the consultation.
9. The practitioner should summarise (reflect back) the story for validation.
10. All information sources should be utilised and documented.

Components of a health history

Identifying data
Identifying data includes the patient's name, age, gender, occupation and marital status. The source of the data should be documented with the date, time and practitioner's signature. This is important as data can be used for referral or previous history elicitation at a later date or for medico-legal reasons.

Presenting complaint
The presenting complaint is the subjective impression formed by the patient of their illness. i.e. 'It hurts when I go to the toilet' or 'I think I may need an x-ray for my foot'. This data is imperative as it forms the basis of the questioning and diagnosis by the practitioner.

History of presenting illness

A clear and chronological account of the problems prompting the patient to seek care should be elicited. This data should include the onset of the problem, the setting in which it occurred and any associated symptoms and treatment action taken at the time by the patient.

Each principal symptom should be documented using the PQRST framework. For example, pain:

P – provocative/palliative or remitting and relieving factors: What makes the pain better, what makes the pain worse?

Q – quality: What is it like, e.g. stabbing, gnawing? How bad is the pain?

R – radiation: If the pain is localised, where else exactly does it hurt? Is the pain referred to anywhere else in the body?

S – site: Where exactly is the focal point of the pain?

T – timing: When did the pain start, was it an acute onset or chronic, has it become worse, is it continuous or intermittent?

Past history

This section is important as it will begin to focus down on any particular illnesses or diseases the patient has experienced in the past and may aid diagnosis. It is appropriate to list all childhood and adult illnesses in each of the areas:

- **Medical**, e.g. diabetes, asthma with dates of onset and hospitalisation.
- **Surgical**, e.g. tonsillectomy, appendectomy with dates, indications and secondary problems experienced as a result of the surgical intervention, e.g. wound infection, wound dehiscence.
- **Obstetric/gynaecological**, e.g. obstetric history, menstrual history, birth control, sexual preference, STD status inclusive of HIV.

Medications

The practitioner should include all prescribed medications and those purchased over the counter and/or alternative therapies used. This can also be used as a medical reinforcement as quite often the patient will indicate that they have no pertinent medical history yet when the professional elicits a drug history, it becomes obvious that they have forgotten to include a specific and sometimes relevant illness, e.g. hypertension or hypercholestereamia.

REFLECTION: Think about certain medications and even drinks that may have interactions with medications you will want to prescribe, e.g. cranberry juice and anticoagulants, levonorgestril and St John's wort.

Allergies

The practitioner should also include a list of allergies to medications. No drug reactions should be written as NKDA (no known drug allergies). Dietary or environment allergies should also be included, e.g. dairy or latex, as this may be pertinent for treatment advice.

Social history

Social history is important as the practitioner will be able to elicit areas of a patient's lifestyle which may be of detriment or associated with the current presenting illness, e.g. employment, accommodation, financial, relationships, appetite, weight, sleep pattern and diurnal variations.

Family history

The age, health and cause of death of each immediate family member including grandparents, parents, siblings and grandchildren should be included with any other relevant disease specific information, e.g. hypertension, coronary artery disease, cancer, mental illness.

Mental health history

Cultural constructs of mental illness vary causing marked differences in acceptance and attitudes. The practitioner should ask open-ended questions initially and be sensitive to reports of mood changes or symptoms such as fatigue, tearfulness, appetite or weight change. If appropriate, suicide risk should be deduced.

A history related to mental health needs should also take into account dependence on alcohol and drugs. The most widely used screening tool is CAGE. Two or more affirmative answers to CAGE may suggest alcohol dependence:

C – Have you ever felt the need to **cut down** on drinking?
A – Have you ever felt **annoyed** by criticism of drinking?
G – Have you ever felt **guilty** about drinking?
E – Have you ever taken a drink first thing in the morning **(eye opener)** to steady your nerves or get rid of a hangover (Mayfield et al., 1974)?

Bates (2007) suggests with alcohol related illnesses it is also pertinent to talk about blackouts (loss of memory of events during drinking), seizures, accidents or injuries while drinking, job loss, marital conflict or legal problems. CAGE can be used to ask similar questions about recreational drugs and certain prescription drugs such as sleeping pills, diet pills and pain killers.

The mini-mental state examination (MMSE, 1975) (see *Box 5.2*) is another useful tool for screening of mental health problems in particular cognitive dysfunction and dementia.

Box 5.2 The mini-mental state examination

Patient _____

Examiner _____

Date _____

Maximum Score

Orientation

5	( )	What is the (year) (season) (date) (day) (month)?
5	( )	Where are we (county) (country) (town) (hospital) (floor)?

Registration

3	( )	Name three objects: 1 second to say each. Then ask the patient all three after you have said them. Give 1 point for each correct answer
		Then repeat them until he/she learns all three. Count trials and record

Trials _____

Attention and calculation

5	( )	Serial 7s. 1 point for each correct answer. Stop after five answers. Alternatively spell 'world' backwards

Recall

3	( )	Ask for the names of the three objects given above. Give 1 point for each correct answer

Language

2	( )	Name a pencil and a watch
1	( )	Repeat the following 'No ifs, ands or buts'

3	( )	Follow a three-stage command: 'Take a paper in your hand, fold it in half and put this on the floor'
1	( )	Read and obey the following: CLOSE YOUR EYES
1	( )	Write a sentence
1	( )	Copy the design shown

Total score _____

Assess level of consciousness along a continuum _____

Alert   Drowsy   Stupor   Coma

(MMSE, 1975)

Sexual and spiritual needs

Sexual and spiritual needs should also be identified and include:

- sexual health (active sexual life, partners, relationships, difficulties, symptoms, if appropriate)
- spiritual health (religion, beliefs, what-who provides a sense of purpose).

Physical assessment

Physical examination is the process by which a health professional investigates the body of a patient for signs and symptoms of disease. It follows the taking of a medical history and aids the correct diagnosis and devising of the treatment plan.

Although professionals have varying approaches to physical examination and there is no right or wrong way to the sequence, a systematic examination generally starts at the head and finishes at the extremities. After the main organ systems relevant to the complaint have been investigated other more specific tests may follow, e.g. a neurological investigation or orthopaedic examination.

With the information obtained during the history and physical examination the practitioner can then formulate an 'impression' or 'differential diagnosis': a list of potential causes of the symptoms. Specific diagnostic tests will then confirm the cause, e.g. blood tests or x-ray.

Internet sites with best practice guidance on disease specific diagnosis and treatment include www.prodigy-nhs.org.uk, www.patient.co.uk and www.nice.org.uk. These websites can be helpful for both patient and professional.

General appearance

The patient's general appearance should be observed as they enter the consultation room. This often elicits a good starting point for the presenting complaint, e.g. mobility problems and gait which may be particularly pertinent if there is a limb problem, dishevelled appearance, weight loss, fatigue or weakness possibly due to illness.

Organ systems

Skin

The practitioner should inspect the patient's skin for rashes, lumps, sores, itching, changes in skin or nails and changes in size or colour of moles. Hair should also be included for symptoms such as baldness, hair loss (alopecia) and differences in texture, distribution and thickness. Inspection of the nails should note colour (cyanosis or pallor), shape (clubbing, indicative of pulmonary, cardiac, familial, systemic, e.g. cirrhosis, ulcerative colitis, coeliac and Crohn's disease) and any lesions (onycholysis, i.e. the painful separation of the nail from the nailbed).

Skin colour should be taken into account, i.e. cyanosis, jaundice, local inflammation and anaemia. Note the skin texture, temperature and moisture content, e.g. dry or oily. The mobility of the skin (ease at which a fold of skin can be moved) and turgor (decreased in dehydration) should also be documented.

Note any lesions and their anatomical location and distribution pattern, shape and type. Grading and description of skin markings should be described as shown in *Box 5.3*.

Box 5.3 Describing and identifying skin markings

- **Bulla**: 1.0 cm or larger and filled with serous fluid, e.g. blistered insect bite
- **Burrow**: raised tunnel in the epidermis commonly found on the webs of the fingers, e.g. scabies
- **Cyst**: nodule filled with expressible material
- **Fissure**: linear crack in the skin often resulting in excessive dryness, e.g. athlete's foot
- **Macule**: small spot up to 1.0 cm
- **Nodule**: marble like lesion larger than 0.5 cm, deeper and firmer than a papule
- **Papule**: up to 1.0 cm
- **Patch**: flat spot 1.0 cm or larger, e.g. café-au-lait spot
- **Plaque**: elevated superficial lesion 1.0 cm or larger, e.g. psoriasis
- **Pustule**: filled with pus, e.g. acne

- **Tumour**: irregular darkened raised area with possible broken skin – evidence of size increase
- **Ulcer**: break to skin with delayed healing time. In lower limbs this may be venous, arterial diabetic, etc. Tests such as Doppler testing will confirm causative illness. Aphthous mouth ulcers can be due to injury, lack of iron, poor health and evidence of stress
- **Vesicle**: up to 1.0 cm filled with serous fluid, e.g. herpes simplex
- **Wheal**: irregular relative transient superficial area of localised oedema, e.g. urticaria

The ABCDE screen is widely used for dysplastic nevi/melanomas:

- **as**ymmetry
- irregular **bo**rders
- variation in **col**our
- **di**ameter > 6mm
- **el**evation (Bates, 2007).

The practitioner should elicit a thorough history of skin changes as specific conditions such as pyoderma gangrenosum, erythema nodosum and acanthosis nigricans may also be associated with specific diseases (ulcerative colitis, sardicosis and polycystic ovary syndrome respectively). Consider *Case studies 5.1* and *5.2*.

Case study 5.1 Phytophotodermatitis

A patient presented after the first initial vesiculobulbous rash had subsided. Hyper pigmentation follows the resolution of the rash. The rash had a bizarre network of geometric streaks. On questioning the woman, she explained that she had been gardening on a sunny day and digging up parsnips and celery. Both these plants contain a chemical that react with ultraviolet light, which causes blistering and pigmentation to those who come into contact with them.

Case study 5.2 Contact dermatitis

While pouring cement from the mixer, Mr H spilt some into his boots. The cement soaked into his socks, which he continued to wear for the rest of the day. Over the following days he developed an itchy rash in the distribution of his socks. Two weeks later there was an excoriated area with marked erythema. The cause: cement, which contains the irritant lime. Advised: new socks, emollient and topical steroids.

Head and neck area

Head

Headache is an extremely common symptom that requires careful evaluation because a small fraction of headaches arise from life-threatening conditions. The practitioner needs to ask about the type of headache and associated symptoms such as nausea and vomiting, changes in vision or smell.

Types of headache include:

- **Migraine**: unilateral headache with associated symptoms such as nausea and photophobia. A migraine can be described with or without aura. Consider *Case study 5.3*.
- **Tension headache**: pain in the scalp, head or neck usually associated with muscle tightness, stress and/or tension.
- **Cluster headache**: unilateral headache that occurs in a cluster effect repeatedly at the same time of the day for several weeks. Tearing of the eye and nasal congestion are also associated with this type of headache.
- **Medication overuse headaches**: pain in the scalp, head or neck usually associated with taking too much analgesia to relieve a headache or pain. One in 50 adults suffers with this (British Association for the Study of Headaches, 2004).
- **Temporal arteritis**: unilateral throbbing headache associated with inflammation or damage to the branches of the external carotid artery in the neck.
- **Sub-arachnoid haemorrhage/aneurysm/intracerebral haemorrhage**: usually described as the 'worst headache in a patient's life' may be associated with decreased mental health and cognitive behaviour, nausea and vomiting. This type of headache may also present with no symptoms. A good family history may aid diagnosis. This is a medical emergency (http://www.nlm.nih.gov/medlineplus (accessed May 2007)).

Case study 5.3 Menstrual migraine

Mrs H suffered from episodic and disabling headaches unilaterally without aura, which were not relieved by regular analgesia. On undertaking a headache diary and cross-referencing the pattern of attacks with the menstrual period, it was found that Mrs H suffered from menstrual migraine, largely related to the fall of oestrogen levels at this time.

Eyes

Disorders of vision tend to increase with age. When checking disorders of the eyes it is pertinent for the practitioner to ascertain any degeneration of visual acuity (VA). Is there a variation from the norm or is visual acuity normal? A snellen chart is used to check acuity using the six metres/six visual acuity metric.

The position and alignment of the eyes and eyebrows should also be noted. Eyelid droop or lag (ptosis) can be a congenital deformity or can be the result of injury or disease, while bacterial infections of the lid can result in the formation of a stye or blephritis. Inspect the sclera and conjunctiva of each eye. Generalised redness without injury may denote conjunctivitis. Assess for diagnosis specific, e.g. allergic or viral (usually bilateral redness) or bacterial infection (usually unilateral). Using oblique lighting inspect the cornea, iris and lens. It may be possible to identify abnormalities such as cataract or iritis.

Compare pupils and test their reactions to light utilising the format PEARRLA: pupils equal and round reacting to light and accommodation.

Lastly, the practitioner should assess the visual fields that may identify defects from diseases such as cerebrovascular accidents (CVA) and the extra-occular movements of the eye using the six cardinal positions of gaze (nystagmus and strabismus may be identified).

Specific tests may require the use of an ophthalmoscope to inspect the fundi for any glaucomatous cupping or disease specific degenerative changes, e.g. haemorrhage or hypertension. The eye may also require staining to rule out foreign body penetration or a corneal abrasion that may later result in ulceration.

Nose and sinuses

The practitioner should examine the external nose using a light and nasal spectum, inspecting the nasal mucosa, septum and turbinates. A viral rhinitis is usually red and swollen while pallor may denote symptoms of allergy especially pertinent in the summer months. The frontal and maxillary sinuses require palpation for tenderness suggestive of sinusitis. This may be concurrent with symptoms of a headache.

Ears

Inspection of the auricle, external acoustic meatus and tympanic membrane will highlight signs of infection, otitis externa or otitis media and will also help diagnose wax impaction and tympanic membrane perforation. Occasionally grommets and grommet insertion scarring can be seen over the tympanic membrane.

The practitioner should also check auditory acuity to ascertain if it is diminished from the norm. If acuity is diminished, lateralisation should be checked using the Weber test (tuning fork to forehead), comparing bone and air conduction and Rinne test (placing the vibrating fork on the mastoid bone and then removing). Both these tests will help differentiate sensorineural hearing loss from conduction problems. Consider *Case study 5.4.*

Case study 5.4 Painful ears

Sean is a 14-year-old boy who has just returned from holiday in Spain. He has been swimming most days in the sea and on the airplane complained of painful ears. Mum had given the child analgesia with nil improvement. He continues to be in pain. He also suffered cold symptoms while he was on holiday:

- What are the differential diagnoses?
- What are you looking for?
- If otitis externa were diagnosed, what would be the treatment?
- What advice would you give to mum?

Mouth and pharynx

Inspection of the lips will highlight issues of central cyanosis. The practitioner should check the oral mucosa for signs of ulceration which may denote ill health and inspect the gums and teeth for dental decay. The tongue, palate, uvula and tonsular pillars should also be inspected and may highlight illnesses such as tonsillitis, quinsy and uvulitis. Hoarseness usually denotes pharyngitis. Tonsillitis should be graded as:

- **grade 1**, visible
- **grade 2**, midway between the tonsular pillars and uvula
- **grade 3**, touching the uvula
- **grade 4**, touching each other (http://www.aafp.org (accessed May 2007)).

Other more specialised tests include a neurological exam of the 12 pairs of cranial nerves, i.e. tongue symmetry: a deviation may denote a CN × 11 paralyses. These tests may elicit problems of a neurological nature.

Neck

The practitioner should inspect and palpate the cervical lymph nodes. Cervical lymphadenopathy will often occur due to an inflammatory response, e.g. tonsillitis, dental abscess. More specialised testing may involve palpation of the supra-clavicular nodes for pathologies relating to the breast, axillae and arm and palpation of the thyroid gland both at rest and when the patient swallows. This is to elicit signs of goitre or thyroiditis.

The practitioner should also note any deviation of the trachea, which may result from a pneumothorax or neck mass.

Breasts, axillae and epitrochlear nodes
Breast tissue should be inspected and palpated for size, symmetry, flattening or contours and oedema (*peu d'orange* – breast cancer). Any nipple inversion or retraction should also be identified noting any discharge or inflammation present. If abnormalities are identified the size, shape and consistency should be documented using the clock format, i.e. 1 cm mass mobile non-tender at 6 o'clock.

The practitioner should palpate the axilliary and epitrochlear nodes for abnormalities in both male and female patients.

Cardiovascular system

The heart is a specialised system and the health professional may need to refer any abnormalities or seek second opinions from the general practitioner or cardiologist.

The practitioner should commence the cardiac examination by measuring the radial and apical pulse and taking the patient's blood pressure. This should be compared with previous readings elicited at earlier dates, if available. Jugular pulsations (bed elevated to 30°) should be observed and the jugular venous pressure (JVP) in relation to the sternal angle recorded. This should normally measure less than three to four cm. An elevated JVP is suggestive of right-sided heart failure, while a decreased JVP can occur in dehydration or a gastrointestinal bleed. Inspection and palpation of the carotid pulsations may elicit bruits, indicative of atherosclerotic narrowing.

The practitioner should inspect and palpate the anterior chest for heaves, lifts or thrills and with the patient turned to the left side the apex of the heart can be examined. This may be displaced due to pregnancy and in left ventricular failure may have an increased impulse diameter. While supine, the rest of the heart can be listened to, e.g. the right ventricular impulse in the parasternal and epigastric areas and thrills noted within the left and right second interspaces.

Auscultation of the heart will illicit S1 and S2 heart sounds and any abnormalities such as aortic regurgitation, murmurs and systolic clicks. The practitioner must describe these in detail, identifying timing in relation to the cardiac cycle, the shape of the sound, e.g. plateau or crescendo, the location of maximal intensity and the radiation, pitch, quality and intensity.

The auscultation assistant at http://www.med.ucla.edu/wilkes/inex.htm is a useful learning aid. This site will enable the practitioner to become competent in different types of heart sound and abnormality.

Lungs

To examine the chest, it is considered best practice to compare left with right and start with the posterior chest wall ending with the anterior.

The practitioner should inspect the thorax observing the shape of the patient's chest, e.g. is it normal or barrel shaped, and note respiratory movements such as symmetrical chest expansion, rate, rhythm depth and effort. Any notable stridors or wheezes should be documented and may be indicative of asthma, COPD or a chest infection.

The chest should be palpated for any areas of tenderness and utilising examination techniques such as tactile fremitus, the professional should be able to pinpoint areas of dullness, e.g. when fluid replaces normal air-filled lungs (infection or mass) or areas of hyper-resonance (emphysema or pneumothorax). Auscultation to all lung fields will further pinpoint areas of abnormality, documented as 'adventitious sounds' not dissipated on coughing, e.g. crackles – fine and coarse. The auscultation assistant (given earlier) also covers lung sounds and abnormalities.

A sudden acute episode of dyspnoea or shortness of breath should be considered a medical emergency if an acute pulmonary embolism is suspected.

Abdomen

The practitioner should utilise the four-quadrant rule (an invisible line drawn through the umbilicus as a centre measure) or the nine-quadrant rule as a framework for examination (see Figure 5.1).

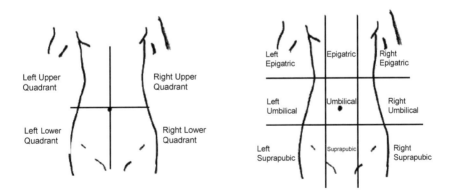

Figure 5.1 Four- and nine-quadrant framework

Four quadrant framework:

- upper left quadrant (ULQ)
- upper right quadrant (URQ)
- lower left quadrant (LLQ)
- lower right quadrant (LRQ).

The examination should also commence furthest away from the site of pain. There are three broadly defined categories of abdominal pain:

- **Visceral pain** (organ pain) described as gnawing, burning and aching. Associated symptoms include nausea, fever, pallor and restlessness, e.g. visceral pain in the right upper quadrant may suggest alcoholic hepatitis.
- **Parietal pain** (inflammation of the peritoneum) described as stabbing and localised, e.g. in an appendicitis periumbilical pain from an inflamed appendix gradually moves from the right lower quadrant to the left lower quadrant.
- **Referred pain**, e.g. biliary tree pain can be referred to the shoulder or right posterior chest.

The practitioner should undertake auscultation before percussion and palpation as both these techniques may increase disturbance and hence sound, which could lead to a false diagnosis. Auscultation can detect hyperresonance and hence increased gastric motility (suggestive of gastroenteritis) and may also elicit bruits from renal or aortic stenosis. Palpation is both light and deep to enable detection of tenderness or inflammation or abnormalities in organs.

Once the abdominal cavity has been examined, further techniques may be used to explore individual organs. If a kidney infection is suspected then both the left and right costovertebral angles (CVA) should be percussed. Tenderness may be suggestive of pylonephritis. Equally Murphy's sign: pressing deeply into the right costal margin at the edge of the rectus muscle and asking the patient to take a deep breath will produce pain with cholecystitis. Cholecystitis usually presents with epigastric pain referred to the back and upper right shoulder margin.

A firm board-like abdominal wall is suggestive of peritoneal inflammation. The patient may lie still and guard the area. Where peritoneal inflammation is suspected rebound tenderness should be checked.

A rectal examination (retroceacal appendicitis) and Rovsing's sign (lower right quadrant pain on pressing deeply and evenly in the left lower right quadrant and quickly withdrawing fingers) can be utilised to detect a possible appendicitis.

Consider *Case study 5.5.*

Case study 5.5 Appendicitis?

Mr P is a 57-year-old working man who is complaining of intermittent heart burn and epigastric pain. This occurs three times a week especially after large or spicy late-night meals. For several years he has been buying over-the-counter antacids and taking them as they relieved his symptoms but now he is experiencing more frequent periods of discomfort:

- What is his diagnosis?
- What treatment and diagnostic investigation should be offered?
- What would be the alarm/red flag symptoms?
- What health promotion advice should you offer?

Children often present with abdominal pains and viral symptoms. Although this is very common, be sure to rule out constipation, appendicitis and urinary tract infections.

Muscular-skeletal system

To identify a musculoskeletal defect GALS (gait, arms, legs and spine), a 10-minute rapid validated screening examination can be utilised. If an abnormality is detected, then a more detailed regional examination must be carried out. This tool developed foremost for general practitioners is now used by medics within the acute sector (Doherty et al., 1992). It is supported for use by the Arthritis Research Campaign (ARC) and more information is available from www.qub.ac.uk/cskills/gals.htm. A summary is detailed in Table 5.1.

Summary

Developing consultation skills and hence the competence to undertake history taking and physical assessment skills takes time and an individual should not expect to have mastered the art of enhanced professional competence without taking time to practise and develop. This may take 12 months to 3 years and the employer should be expected to support the professional through this period of learning. This period of learning should be accepted by the professional as a period of reflection as it is should be remembered that in accordance with the Nursing and Midwifery Council's Code, standards of

Table 5.1 Summary of GALS assessment: gait, arms legs spine

Screening questions for musculoskeletal disorders
1 Do you have any pain or stiffness in your arms, legs or back?
2 Can you walk up and down stairs without difficulty?
3 Can you dress yourself in everyday clothes without any difficulty?

Screening examination for musculoskeletal disorders

Gait	Ask the patient to walk a few steps, turn & walk back.	Observe the patients gait for symmetry, smoothness and the ability to turn quickly.
	With the patient in the anatomical position, inspect from the posterior, lateral and anterior aspects.	Observe for any abnormalities in the muscles (e.g. reduced muscle bulk), spine (e.g. abnormal spinal curvature such as scoliosis), limbs or joints (e.g. a red swollen knee)
Spine	Inspection	Inspect the spine for any abnormalities including abnormal kyphosis, scolosis or loss of lordosis.
	Neck movements	Ask the patient to tilt their head to each side, bringing the ear towards their shoulder. Assess the degree of lateral neck flexion.
	Lumbar spine movement	Ask the patient to bend forward and touch their toes. During this movement the patient may depend partly on good hip flexion to bend forwards. So it is always a good idea to palpate for the range of lumbar movement. Place two fingers over the lumbar vertebra. As the patient bends forward your fingers should move apart (assuming the patient has a good range of lumbar spine movement).
Arms	Shoulder movements	Ask the patient to place their hands behind their head, with their elbows back This movement assesses abduction, external rotation of the shoulder and elbow flexion.
	Elbow movements & hands	Ask the patient to extend their arms fully and turn their hands over so palms are down.
		Following this ask the patient to turn their hands over.
		Observe the hands for any joint swelling or deformities.
	Grip strength	Ask the patient to make a fist. Observe the hand and finger movements.

		Ask the patient to grip your fingers and assess the degree of grip strength.
	Precision pinch	Ask the patient to bring each finger in turn to meet the thumb.
	Metacarpalphalangeal squeeze test	Squeeze across the metacarpalphalangeal joints (tenderness here may indicates synovitis of metacarpalphalangeal joints).
Leg	Knee movements	With the patient lying on the couch assess flexion and extension of both knees. Make sure to palpate the knee for crepitus.
	Hip movement	Hold the knee & hip flexed to 90 degrees. Now assess the degree of internal rotation in each hip.
	Patellar tap test	Perform a patellar tap in each knee for the presence of an effusion.
	Inspection of feet	Inspect the feet for any swelling, deformity or any callosities.
	Metacarpalphalangeal squeeze test	Squeeze across the metatarsophalangeal joints for any tenderness.

Record		
	Record your findings	*Mr N Flanders* *21/8/06* *DOB 16/12/1960* *3pm*

Mr N Flanders　　　　　　　　　*21/8/06*
DOB 16/12/1960　　　　　　　　*3pm*

	Appearance	*Movement*
Gait	✓	✓
Arms	✗	✗
Legs	✓	✓
Spine	✓	✓

Suffering over MCP points tender to squeeze – early RAP

Dr B Simpson

conduct, performance and ethics a nurse is personally accountable for actions or omissions and must always be able to justify their decisions.

Defined by Epstein and Hundert (2002), professional competence is the habitual and judicious use of communication, knowledge, technical skills, clinical reasoning, emotions, values and reflection in daily practice for the benefit of the individual and the community being served. Through the development of first contact and complex needs assessment skills advanced primary care professionals can enhance provision of care for patients.

References

Aggleton, P. and Chalmers, H. (2000) *Nursing Models and Nursing Practice*, 2nd edn. London, Macmillan.

Baird, A. (2001) Diagnosis and prescribing. *Primary Health Care* 11, 5, 24–26.

Bates, B. (1995) *A Guide to Physical Examination and History Taking*, 6th edn. Philadelphia, PA, J.B. Lippincott Company.

Bates, B. (2007) *Pocket Guide to Physical Examination*, 5th edn. Philadelphia, PA, J.B. Lippincott Company.

British Association for the Study of Headache (2004) *Guidelines for All Doctors in the Diagnosis and Management of Migraine and Tension-type Headache*. London, British Association for the Study of Headache.

Byrne, P. S. and Long, B. (1976) *Doctors Talking to Patients*. London, HMSO.

Doherty, M., Dacre, J., Dieppe, P. and Snaith, M. (1992) The 'GALS' locomotor screen. *Annals of the Rheumatic Diseases* 51, 1165–1169.

Epstein, R. and Hundert, E. (2002) Defining and assessing professional competence. *Journal of the American Medical Association* 287, 226–235.

Mayfield, D., McLeod, G. and Hall, P. (1974) The CAGE questionnaire: validation of a new alcoholism instrument. *American Journal of Psychiatry* 131, 1121–1123.

MMSE (1975) Mini-mental state: a practical method for grading the cognitive state of patients for the clinician. *Journal of Psychiatric Research* 12, 3, 189–198.

Nursing and Midwifery Council (2008) The Code. Standards of conduct, performance and ethics for nurses and midwives. London, NMC.

Pendleton, D., Schofield, T., Tate, P. and Havelock, P. (1984) *The Consultation: an approach to learning and teaching*. Oxford, Oxford University Press.

Ramsey, P. G., Curtis, J. R., Paauw, D. S., Carline, J. D. and Wenrich, M. D. (1998) History taking and preventative medicine skills among primary care physicians: an assessment using standardised patients. *American Journal of Medicine* 104, 2, 152–158.

Royal College of Nursing (RCN) (2004) *Nurse Practitioners: an RCN guide to the nurse practitioner role, competences and programme*. London, RCN.

Silverman, J., Kurtz, S. and Draper, J. (1998) *Skills for Communicating with Patients*. Oxford, Radcliffe Medical Press.

Stott, N. and Davies, R (1979) The exceptional potential in each primary care consultation. *Journal of the Royal College of General Practitioners* 29, 210–216.

http://www.aafp.org (accessed 05/2007).

http://www.med.ucla.edu/wilkes/inex.htm (accessed 05/2007).

http://www.nlm.nih.gov/medlineplus (accessed 05/2007).

http://www.qub.ac.uk/cskills/gals.htm (accessed 08/2007).

6 Non-medical prescribing

Virginia Radcliffe

Introduction

Advanced primary care nurses often are the first contact for the public in the healthcare system and may be the only contact for patients with the NHS. For practitioners in advanced practice roles, prescribing is an enhanced skill that is vital for comprehensive patient care. If advanced primary care practitioners are able to diagnose and prescribe autonomously, then waiting times could be reduced, patients will have improved access to medicines and patient care and safety can be improved. This chapter will outline the context of non-medical prescribing and the professional, legal and practical considerations for advanced primary care practitioners.

Context of non-medical prescribing

The Cumberlege Report (*Neighbourhood Nursing: a focus for care*) (DHSS, 1986) recommended that community nurses with a district nurse (DN) or health visitor (HV) specialist practice qualification have limited prescribing rights. It was identified that patient care could be improved and the use of resources be used more effectively if nurses were able to prescribe those items that were within their usual scope of practice and expertise. The government commissioned the Advisory Group on Nurse Prescribing, chaired by Dr June Crown, to review the findings of the Cumberlege Report. The Crown Report (DH, 1989) recommended the introduction of prescribing by selected nurses from a *Nurses' Formulary*. This report recommended the categories of items that nurses might prescribe such as simple analgesia, wound, catheter and bowel management products, the circumstances for prescribing those items, as well as the legislative, funding and training requirements.

In 1992, the primary legislation Medicinal Products; Prescription by Nurses' Act was passed, which extended the prescribing rights to DNs and HVs who have undergone further training, a legal right to prescribe specific products. By 1994, eight demonstration sites were established, the *Nurse Prescribers' Formulary* (NPF) (NPF, 2005) was produced and the secondary legislation Medicinal Prescription by Nurses etc. (Commencement No. 1)

Order came into effect. The pilots were successful and demonstrated that nurse prescribing improved patient care; enhanced professional responsibility for the nurses involved; and reduced the workload for general practitioners (Luker et al., 1997, 1998). Nurse prescribing (V100) was rolled out and by 2001 over 20,000 DNs and HVs were qualified prescribers and the training was incorporated into the specialist practitioner qualification for DNs and HVs.

In 2005 the NPF became the NPF for Community Practitioners (NPF, 2005) and all specialist community practitioners (district nurses, health visitors/specialist community public health nurses, school nurses, community mental health nurses, learning disabilities nurses, occupational health nurses, practice nurses and children's community nurses) are eligible to undertake nurse prescribing (V100) as part of their specialist practitioner qualification provided they intend to practise in an area of clinical need for which prescribing from the NPF will improve patient care (Nursing and Midwifery Council (NMC), 2006a).

In 1999 a second report by Crown (DH, 1999) reviewed the prescribing, supply and administration of medicines. This review recommended that prescribing rights be extended to other professional groups with training and expertise in specialist areas. Support from government was granted (DH, 2001a) and funding was provided for the training programme to allow nurses to prescribe from an extended formulary. The *Extended Nurse Prescribers' Formulary* (ENPF) included all general sales list (GSL) medicines, all licensed pharmacy (P) medicines and 140 prescription-only medicines (POMs) which could only be prescribed for specified conditions under four categories, i.e. minor illness, minor injury, health promotion and palliative care. In 2003, the ENPF was expanded to include additional conditions and medicines, including some controlled drugs. However, the ENPF remained restrictive and did not meet the needs of many specialist practitioners.

Independent prescribing

Following a wide consultation process (DH, 2005a), the *Nurse Prescribers' Extended Formulary* was discontinued on 1 May 2006. Qualified nurse independent prescribers (formerly known as extended formulary nurse prescribers) are now able to prescribe any licensed medicine for any medical condition within their scope of practice and competence, including some controlled drugs (DH, 2006a). Pharmacists can now also become independent prescribers and they have the same prescribing rights as nurse independent prescribers within their own level of experience and competence and in accordance with Royal Pharmaceutical Society of Great Britain (RPSGB) guidance (RPSGB, 2006).

Independent nurse prescribers are able to prescribe medicines outside the terms of their licence (off label). Off-label prescribing is prescribing a medicine that is licensed for a particular set of indications but is used for another. There are a number of circumstances when nurses may prescribe off label such as when prescribing for children or for palliative care. The prescriber must ensure they are satisfied there is sufficient evidence to demonstrate the medicine's safety and no alternative licensed medicine is available before prescribing (NMC, 2006a).

In the United Kingdom, an unlicensed medicine is one that does not have a license from the Medicines Control Agency (MCA) and can only be prescribed by supplementary prescribers under a clinical management plan (CMP). Unlicensed and off-label medicines should only be used where there is no suitable licensed alternative. If practitioners wish to prescribe controlled drugs or unlicensed medicines (as part of a clinical drugs trial), or widen their scope of practice, then supplementary prescribing can facilitate this.

Supplementary prescribing

Supplementary prescribing was first termed dependent prescribing by Crown (DH, 1999) and was introduced in 2003 for nurses and pharmacists (DH, 2003). In 2005 physiotherapists, podiatrist, radiographers and optometrists were added (DH, 2005b). Supplementary prescribing is a formal partnership between an independent prescriber (who must be a doctor or dentist in this instance) and the supplementary prescriber(s) to implement an agreed patient-specific clinical management plan (CMP) and can only take place once the independent prescriber has made a diagnosis (DH, 2003). The CMP must include details of the condition(s) to be treated, the class or description of medicines that can be prescribed and the circumstances in which the supplementary prescriber should refer to or seek advice from the doctor/dentist. The details of the medicines can be as specific or broad as the supplementary prescriber requires. For example, an experienced diabetes podiatrist might specify the National Service Framework for Diabetes (DH, 2001b) as the details of the medicines, whereas a practice nurse who has recently begun managing asthma patients in the practice may require specific guidance on the individual medicines to prescribe, including dosage ranges.

Supplementary prescribers must have access to the same patient/client health records as the doctor/dentist and access to a prescribing budget. There are no legal restrictions on the clinical conditions for which supplementary prescribers can prescribe (DH, 2005b). All medicines can be prescribed once specified in the CMP including controlled drugs and unlicensed medicines; if they are part of a clinical drugs trial with a clinical trial certificate.

It is impractical to use supplementary prescribing for one-off prescribing as the diagnosis must be established by a doctor and a CMP must be in place before the supplementary prescriber can prescribe. However, supplementary prescribing lends itself to the management of long-term conditions or ongoing prescribing very well. More than one supplementary prescriber can be included on each CMP and so it is useful for team prescribing to ensure continuity of care. It is an excellent method of prescribing in areas where the prescriber is less confident as the CMP can provide detailed prescribing guidance. Nurses and pharmacists might use supplementary prescribing when newly qualified as a prescriber or if widening their scope of practice. Allied health professionals may only prescribe using supplementary prescribing and so need to identify how this would work in their clinical practice.

Patient group directions

Patient group directions (PGDs) are written instructions for the supply and/or administration of a named medicine(s) in an identified clinical situation. Therefore, PGDs are *not* a form of prescribing but a method of supplying and/ or administering medicines. There are no specific training requirements for health professionals to complete before using PGDs, although individual organisations have a responsibility to ensure those who use them are competent to do so. Many healthcare professionals are eligible to use PGDs, including nurses, ambulance paramedics, physiotherapists and pharmacists. PGDs were first identified by Crown (DH, 1999) and were predominately devised for large-group prescribing such as immunisation campaigns. Many trusts have embraced PGDs as they do not require staff to undertake a lengthy training programme and can be used by many practitioners at once. PGDs are suitable to be used in instances when immediate administration of medicines is necessary without having to wait to consult a prescriber or waiting for a prescriber to see the patient. However, they do have their constraints as the patient must fit exactly within the detailed criteria provided for each PGD and they are often complex to develop. They must be ratified through the organisation's clinical governance system and a senior doctor and pharmacist must provide signed authorisation for each PGD.

As a dispensing pharmacist is not involved to check and monitor the medicines when PGDs are used, practitioners must ensure that they are competent to use them safely. Patient safety is paramount and practitioners should refer to the National Prescribing Centre (NPC) guidance for additional information (NPC, 2004). Practitioners need to identify whether the use of PGDs is the safest and most appropriate way for their patients to receive their medicines and seek appropriate training and support. For more information, see *Medicine Matters: a guide to mechanisms to prescribing, supply and administration of medicines* (DH, 2006b).

Legal aspects of prescribing

The law relating to the licensing, prescribing, administration and supply of medicines is detailed in the Medicines Act (1968). Medicines are classified into three categories:

- **prescription-only medicines** (PoMs), which may be supplied, sold or administered against a signed and dated prescription issued by an appropriate practitioner
- **pharmacy-only medicines** (Ps) may be purchased from a registered primary care pharmacy, provided that the pharmacist supervises the sale. Examples include senna tablets and Clotrimazole 1% cream
- **general sales list medicines** (GSL) need neither a prescription nor the supervision of a pharmacist and can be obtained from retail outlets. Examples include paracetamol or cough mixture.

The Misuse of Drugs Act (1971) controls the manufacture, supply and possession of controlled drugs. The penalties relate to the harmfulness of the drug when misused and are categorised into three classes (BNF, 2007):

- **Class A** includes cocaine, opium and morphine
- **Class B** includes oral amphetamines and barbiturates
- **Class C** includes anabolic steroids and most benzodiazepines

The Misuse of Drugs Regulations (2001) defines the classes of person who are authorised to supply and possess controlled drugs within their professional capacity. The regulations specify the requirements controlling activities which include import/export, possession, prescribing and the record keeping which applies to these drugs. They are divided into five schedules:

1 **Schedule 1** includes drugs that are not used medicinally.
2 **Schedule 2** includes morphine and cocaine and are subject to full, controlled drug regulations such as keeping of registers and safe custody.
3 **Schedule 3** includes some barbiturates and are subject to special prescription requirements but not safe custody or registers.
4 **Schedule 4** includes anabolic steroids but controlled drug requirements do not apply.
5 **Schedule 5** includes those preparations that are low in strength and are exempt for virtually all controlled drug requirements.

There are additional prescribing requirements for controlled drugs and pharmacists are not allowed to dispense a controlled drug unless the prescription includes all the information required by law (BNF, 2007).

Preparation for the role of prescriber

Most practitioners undertaking a non-medical prescribing course are funded by the NHS (DH, 2006a). Funding is limited and can be obtained via the prescribing lead for their organization or the strategic health authority. Nurses must provide evidence that they have met the Nursing and Midwifery Council's eligibility criteria (NMC, 2006a). The RPSGB (2006) and the Health Professions Council (HPC, 2007) have similar criteria. Applicants must identify a service need, have the support of their employer and meet the academic requirements of the higher education institution to which they intend to apply. They must also identify a designated medical practitioner who meets the National Prescribing Centre's eligibility criteria (NPC, 2005) and who has agreed to provide the required period of supervised practice. The professional bodies (NMC, RPSGB and HPC) have specified the structure and nature of the education programme. The content includes the legal, professional and ethical aspects of prescribing as well as the consultation process and clinical pharmacology (NPC, 2001, 2003a, 2003b, 2003c).

Courses are part time and are usually delivered over a three-month period consisting of at least 26 taught days and 12 supervised learning-in-practice days. Distance-learning courses must include at least eight face-to-face taught days and 10 days protected learning time, in addition to the 12 days supervised learning in practice (NMC, 2006a). Competence in prescribing is demonstrated through an assessment of theory and practice. This usually involves a written examination, a clinical skills examination and a portfolio of evidence. The independent and supplementary prescribing for nurses' assessments must consist of a written examination with 20 short answer and multi-choice questions to test pharmacological knowledge and its application to practise with an 80% pass mark. There must be satisfactory evidence of completion of practice, competence in numeracy and drug calculations (100% pass mark), prescription writing and prescribing in a range of scenarios (NMC, 2006a). Many prescribing courses are taught inter-professionally, which has added value and improved professional relationships for those involved (Radcliffe, 2006).

The prescribing process

A holistic assessment incorporating a detailed history and physical examination is essential before prescribing for any patient. Practitioners must be competent to diagnose, undertake a history and carry out a clinical assessment in their area of speciality before undertaking a preparation programme to prescribe (NMC, 2006a). In order to complete a holistic assessment successfully, practitioners must have effective patient-centred communication and have gained consent. Consent must be free, full and reasonably informed (Dimond, 2002).

In order to prescribe safely and systematically, the practitioner should identify and use a specific model of consultation such as Neighbour (2004). Roger Neighbour identifies five check points in the patient–practitioner consultation:

- **connecting**: establishing a rapport with the patient
- **summarising**: identifying why the patient has sought advice, listening and obtaining information
- **handing over**: a mutual agreement, negotiation and decision making
- **safety netting**: ensuring all the key points have been identified, record keeping, review and reflection
- **housekeeping**: ensuring that the practitioner is okay to see the next patient.

Once a holistic assessment has been completed, the practitioner can establish what the treatment options are, whether a prescription is appropriate and whether they are competent to prescribe that prescription. If a prescription is necessary, then the practitioner must choose an appropriate medicine. Practitioners must consider the effectiveness, appropriateness, safety, and cost effectiveness of the medicines that they intend to prescribe (NPC, 1999). Prescribers should familiarise themselves with the medicines they intend to prescribe and the supporting clinical evidence available, to ensure evidence-based prescribing. In order to achieve concordance, the medicine, possible side-effects, duration of treatment and expected outcomes should be discussed with the patient and their agreement to take the prescribed medicines must be obtained.

Once these steps have been completed, the practitioner can write the prescription. Prescriptions should be written, dated and signed in indelible ink. The full name and address of the patient/client should be included and the date of birth and age. It is a legal requirement to state the age of a child under 12 years old for a prescription for a PoM. The generic name (where possible) should be written as well as the strength (if applicable), formulation, dosage, frequency, quantity, directions for use and duration of the medicine. For further guidance on prescription writing, see the BNF (2007).

NHS prescriptions can be computer generated, although many non-medical prescribers do not have access to the appropriate software. NHS prescriptions for primary care nurses are lilac-coloured FP10P forms marked *Nurse Independent/Supplementary Prescriber* and are obtained from the trust prescribing lead. Ensure that a specimen of the prescribers' signatures are held by the trust lead and provide one to the local pharmacies who might be dispensing prescriptions, too. Practitioners that will normally have their prescriptions dispensed by hospital pharmacies will use a locally agreed form. Independent prescribers can also issue private prescriptions for any licensed medicine provided that it is within their competency (NMC, 2006a).

Once the prescription has been completed, the assessment must be documented in the patient record. These must be contemporaneous, accurate and detailed in accordance with the professional bodies' guidelines (RSPGB, NMC and IIPC). When a prescription has been written, the GP should be informed within a locally agreed timescale, usually 48 hours. The practitioner should negotiate with the patient whether a follow-up or review is necessary and identify where they can seek advice before the review if needed. Regular monitoring of the patient may include questions about side-effects of the medicine, the effectiveness of the medicine and concordance. Reflecting on prescribing decisions is an important part of the prescribing process and can help practitioners improve and develop their prescribing practice. A reflective diary that documents prescribing decisions and experiences can be a useful approach to evaluate learning.

Professional considerations

All prescribers are professionally responsible for their own actions and omissions. Practitioners are personally accountable for each prescription that they write and their decision to prescribe. Prescribers should not be influenced by others to prescribe, e.g. pharmaceutical representatives, peers, or colleagues. Practitioners must only prescribe within their competence and only if they have assessed the patient. They must only prescribe where there is a genuine need for treatment (NMC, 2006a).

Where a practitioner is appropriately trained and qualified as a prescriber, and prescribes as part of their clinical duties with the consent of the employer, the employer may also be held vicariously liable for negligent acts of their employees committed in the course of their employment. If the practitioner chooses to act outside the scope of their employment, their employer is exempt from liability. Simply because the employer may be vicariously liable does not provide a defence. You are also primarily liable and you may be sued as well. If your employer pays a claim as a result of negligence, they may claim against you for any loss suffered under your employment contract. It is important to ensure that your job description is amended to include prescribing and identify that your trust has a prescribing policy or guidelines in place. It is advisable that all prescribers have professional indemnity insurance through membership of a professional organisation or trade union.

Maintaining competency, once qualified as a prescriber, is the prescriber's own responsibility. Practitioners must remain up to date with the knowledge and skills to enable them to prescribe competently and safely. This includes the developments in prescribing practices and changes to legislation or policy. Employers have a responsibility to ensure that practitioners have access to relevant continuing professional development (CPD) through the staff appraisal system (NMC, 2006a). The NPC (2001, 2003a, 2003b, 2003c) has produced competencies frameworks to assist the practitioner to reflect on their prescribing practice.

Reflection is an essential way to evaluate prescribing. Clinical supervision can enable practitioners to develop competence, improve knowledge, take responsibility for their own practice and enhance patient safety in complex situations. Primary care practitioners have access to prescription analysis and cost tabulation (PACT) data, which summarises the medicines and appliances prescribed over the past three months. The data includes cost comparisons shown both locally and nationally.

The future of non-medical prescribing

Non-medical prescribing has developed rapidly in the last few years in conjunction with the structure of the NHS and the healthcare professionals that work within it. Many pharmacists will now be able to train as independent prescribers following the changes to legislation (DH, 2006a). There are clear advantages for patients who will have improved access to a wider range of medicines. However, there are financial implications such as payment for the work done and the reimbursement of any costs incurred that community pharmacists who prescribe need to resolve.

It is possible that prescribing may eventually be integrated into pre-registration curricula. Staff nurses are now able to prescribe from the NPF for community practitioners after successfully completing a shortened version of the existing independent and supplementary prescribing for nurses course (VISO) (NMC, 2006b). They will need to identify a service need and meet the eligibility requirements set by the NMC. They will need to be supervised in practice by a suitably qualified prescriber and pharmacists and nurses will be able to fulfil this role. This will alleviate some of the difficulties that practitioners have experienced in obtaining a medical practitioner to support them in practice, compounded by the lack of financial remuneration. It is not anticipated that doctors will no longer be mandatory supervisors for other non-medical prescribing courses.

Summary

The fact many healthcare professions are now able to prescribe has widened the public's access to medicines. Practitioners are able to diagnose, prescribe for and maintain a variety of clinical conditions independently, which has given the workforce flexibility and autonomy. Developing this enhanced skill is vital for advanced primary care nurses to practise in an ever-changing health service and meet the health needs of the population.

[Note that the London Metropolitan University Prescribing website offers practitioners opportunities to rehearse prescribing skills and knowledge. www.prescribing.info]

References

British National Formulary (BNF) (2007) *British National Formulary*. London, British Medical Association, Royal Pharmaceutical Society of Great Britain.

Department of Health (DH) (1989) *Report of the Advisory Group on Nurse Prescribing (Crown Report)*. London, DH.

Department of Health (DH) (1999) *Review of Prescribing, Supply and Administration of Medicines (Crown Report 2)*. London, DH.

Department of Health (DH) (2001a) *Patients Get Quicker Access to Medicines. Press release 2001/0223*. London, DH.

Department of Health (DH) (2001b) *National Service Framework for Diabetes: standards*. London, DH.

Department of Health (DH) (2003) *Supplementary Prescribing by Nurses and Pharmacists within the NHS in England: a guide for implementation*. London, DH.

Department of Health (DH) (2005a) *Consultation on Options for the Future of Independent Prescribing by Extended Formulary Nurse Prescribers*. London, DH/MHRA.

Department of Health (DH) (2005b) *Supplementary Prescribing by Nurses, Pharmacists, Chiropodists/Podiatrists, Physiotherapists and Radiographers within the NHS in England: a guide for implementation*. London, DH.

Department of Health (DH) (2006a) *Improving Access to Medicines: a guide to implementing nurse and pharmacist independent prescribing within the NHS in England*. London, DH.

Department of Health (DH) (2006b) *Medicine Matters: a guide to mechanisms to prescribing, supply and administration of medicines.* London, DH.

Department of Health & Social Security (DHSS) (1986) *Neighbourhood Nursing: a focus for care (Cumberlege Report).* London, HMSO.

Dimond, B. (2002) *Legal Aspects of Consent.* Salisbury, Quay Books. Health Professions Council (HPC) (2007) *Standards of Conduct, Performance and Ethics.* London, HPC.

Luker, K., Austin, L., Ferguson, B. and Smith, K. (1997) Nurse prescribing: the views of nurses and other healthcare professionals. *British Journal of Community Nursing* 2, 69–74.

Luker, K. A., Austin, L., Hogg, C., Ferguson, B. and Smith, K. (1998) Nurse-patient relationships: the context of nurse prescribing. *Journal of Advanced Nursing* 28, 2, 235–242.

National Prescribing Centre (NPC) (1999) Seven principles of good prescribing – a step-wise approach. *Prescribing Nurse Bulletin* 1, 1. Liverpool, NPC.

National Prescribing Centre (NPC) (2001) *Maintaining Competency in Prescribing: an outline framework to help nurse prescribers.* Liverpool, NPC.

National Prescribing Centre (NPC) (2003a) *Maintaining Competency in Prescribing: an outline framework to help allied health professional supplementary prescribers.* Liverpool, NPC.

National Prescribing Centre (NPC) (2003b) *Maintaining Competency in Prescribing: an outline framework to help nurse supplementary prescribers.* Liverpool, NPC.

National Prescribing Centre (NPC) (2003c) *Maintaining Competency in Prescribing: an outline framework to help pharmacist supplementary prescribers.* Liverpool, NPC.

National Prescribing Centre (NPC) (2004) *A Practical Guide and Framework of Competencies for All Professionals using Patient Group Directions.* Liverpool, NPC.

National Prescribing Centre (NPC) (2005) *Training Non-Medical Prescribers in Practice: a guide to help doctors prepare for and carry out the role of designated medical practitioner.* Liverpool, NPC.

Neighbour, R. (2004) *The Inner Consultation: how to develop an effective and intuitive consulting style.* Oxford, Radcliffe Publishing.

Nursing and Midwifery Council (NMC) (2006a) *Standards of Proficiency for Nurse and Midwife Prescribers.* London, NMC.

Nursing and Midwifery Council (NMC) (2006b) *Circular 19/2006.* London, NMC.

Radcliffe, V. (2006) *Inter-professional Approaches to Prescribing* (unpublished report). London, London Metropolitan University.

Royal Pharmaceutical Society of Great Britain (RPSGB) (2006) *Medicines, Ethics and Practice – a guide for pharmacists.* London, RPSGB.

PART 3
ENHANCING STRATEGIC SKILLS

7 Developing whole systems thinking

Paul Thomas and Deirdre Kelley-Patterson

Introduction

Whole system thinking means seeing beyond immediate problems to see other things that are relevant to a good outcome – you see your daily work in a bigger picture. As an advanced practitioner you will often need to do this for your patients. As a leader of service developments you will also need to apply a similar approach. For this reason, we have linked this chapter with the next chapter, on transformational leadership.

In this chapter, you will learn a way to think systematically about a whole system. You will learn how to relate discrete focused situations to bigger contexts. And, by way of contrast you will have a way to examine the practical implications of big picture policy change to your day-to-day work. Both these situations involve four stages:

1 **Identify the breadth of issues involved**. You can undertake a rapid appraisal, brainstorm or mapping exercise to reveal the large number of things that impact on everyday situations. Often these factors are quiet and hidden. But when something changes, they can suddenly reveal themselves to either help or hinder a good outcome.
2 **Hold the story**. As an advocate for patients you must help them to tell their stories with all their humanity and complexity – this helps to understand why some ways forward are better than others.
3 **Plan coordinated changes**. When planning future care for a patient or when planning new services, several things will need to change at the same time. Force field analysis, multipurpose databases, backwards mapping and good teams all help to reveal the best ways to bring everyone along together.
4 **Maintain personal balance**. Thinking at so many different levels and appreciating the contributions of so many different people can leave you unsure about who you are – you can feel torn in many directions. Techniques such as visualisation, role play and team working can help you to remain balanced even when multiple forces threaten to knock you over.

The chapter has two sections. The first is concerned with the theory of whole systems thinking, which includes theories about connections. We remind you of the complexities you have to deal with in everyday situations and how they influence one another, both as a practitioner and as a leader of policy for change. We also give an overview of where whole systems thinking came from and where you can read more about it. The second section includes techniques and exercises to help you to improve your skills in these four areas.

Both theory and practical sections are adapted from Thomas (2006).

Theory of whole systems thinking and practice

Consider your role when working with a patient who is dying. Death is a powerful case study because the complexities are easy to imagine and because the consequences of managing it well or badly are immediately obvious. However, the principles are the same for all complex situations including long-term conditions.

When working with a dying patient

Managing a death well is one of the most satisfying tasks of a healthcare professional. It is a high-level skill and involves a lot of hard work. By helping a patient to feel in control of the process and reconciled to it, you can help make it a healthy death. The aim should be that dignity is maintained and the end becomes a celebration of their completed life. He or she must have the right information at the right time, hold on to a coherent life story, have things well planned and find ways to be internally balanced.

There is a breadth of things to consider – where and how to die, who to inform and when, funeral arrangements, financial affairs and the will. The dying person is not the only one to consider – family, friends, neighbours will also be affected and may need your help. You do your job well when you help your patient to gently surface the various things that matter, giving them choice about what they want to do. You do your job well when you *identify the breadth of issues* involved.

Facing death is emotionally difficult for everyone involved. A healthy person has a coherent life story and death can seem very fragmenting. An advanced practitioner must help a patient to see and value the coherence of their life story and rectify whatever they can within it that works against this coherence. Now is the time to remember the good things of the past, to reconcile unnecessary conflicts, and build relationships with those who will be a companion during the final stages. You can help your patient reminisce about their life, supporting them to value the good and face up to regrets and unfinished business. You do your job well when you *help your patient to hold the story*.

There are many things that need to be planned. Through lack of planning someone may be admitted to hospital to die, quite against their wishes and those of their carers. Conversely, when intentions have been discussed and understood, and the plan written down, it is easier to remain faithful to the desired end. Who will be invited to the funeral? What ceremony, music, speeches? Lack of planning makes it difficult for family who are being asked to be creative at a very difficult emotional time for them. You do your job well when you help your patient to *plan coordinated change*.

Even when a death is managed perfectly it is personally confronting for everyone involved. As an advanced practitioner, you need to handle the effect on yourself, and help your patient and carers to do the same. You do your job well when you help all involved to *maintain personal balance*.

When leading policy development for healthy dying

Patients are seen by many general and specialist medical practitioners, as well as out-of-hours doctors and nurses, social workers, voluntary workers, carers, church workers and so on. Good policy includes a system that helps all of these to communicate well with one another when they need to solve a problem and also when developing new services. Good policy also encourages mutual respect and understanding.

There are many things to consider – patient-held records and a reliable way to update these, roles and responsibilities of different disciplines, an agreed way to hand over to night-time services and expected standards of care in a crisis, audit of the system and feedback to all involved. When leading policy change you do your job well when you *identify the breadth of issues involved*.

Within the extended network of people, agencies and issues involved there will be many different interpretations of what are the goals – medical management of symptoms, sensitive management of emotions, managing practical problems, accurate death diagnosis and whether a coroner needs to be informed. Misunderstandings and inefficiencies can be avoided by having a shared understanding of what you are trying to achieve together and your complementary roles to achieve this. You do your job well when you help all involved to *hold the story*.

Coordinated plans are essential in good policy for healthy dying. If one agency tries to do it on its own it will fail and also become increasingly frustrated by the failure of others to do their bit. Synchronous pilot testing of coordinated plans is needed, with ongoing feedback at subsequent meetings to identify glitches in the system. A clear communication system is needed and times when various agencies can come together to review existing services and plan new developments. You do your job well when you help the various agencies involved to *plan coordinated changes.*

Misunderstandings and a sense of chaos are easy to develop when many different people and organisations are involved. Policy needs to systematically build trusted relationships to help avoid these, as well as safe spaces to talk things through and ways to support those who have felt unappreciated. These are all concerned with helping all involved to remain confident and balanced, wanting to continue to contribute to the quality of the whole system. You do your job well when you help all involved to *maintain personal balance.*

These examples of patient care and policy development just given show how these four, apparently simple stages help us make sense of complexity. When increasing numbers of overlapping systems and people are involved, it becomes increasingly difficult to keep track of everything. In the next chapter, on transformational leadership, we help you to use these same four stages on a larger stage.

Consider *Case study 7.1.*

Case study 7.1 Making sense of complexity

A general practice out-of-hours service sought to understand why patients who expressed a desire to die at home were sometimes admitted to die in hospital. A rapid appraisal revealed a large number of projects exploring the same concern, unaware of one another. Key informants, including leaders of these various projects, were invited to take part in a workshop where they role played different perspectives. This revealed that each individual was doing their best, but was trapped by the system. The 'patients' perceived that the visiting doctor did not know patient wishes, the 'out-of-hours doctors' claimed that they were not given information by the daytime doctors and the 'in-hours doctors' said that there was no overall leadership to develop a better communication system. They drew a diagram that showed how the efforts of everyone are interdependent and success requires coordinated interdisciplinary communication. A cross-organisational team was formed to provide shared leadership for change. They wrote a revised diagram, more able to support good communication. This required simultaneous changes in the policy of different organisations. At a whole system event, senior members from these organisations agreed to pilot these changes. Repeated cycles of piloting and learning from data emerging from the pilots produced a better system of whole system communication with an inbuilt mechanism for ongoing evaluation.

Whole systems theory – hard, soft and complex adaptive systems

There are many different schools of thought about systems. The traditional idea of a *hard system* is a linear set of links in a chain. The cardiovascular system is an example – the heart pumps blood one way through a set of arteries and back through veins that go back to the heart. The idea of a *soft system* is described by Checkland (1995). Multiple nutrients crossing a cell wall of a heart muscle is an example – multiple chemicals compete and collaborate together and are dependent on the exact situation. A *whole system* has been described by Pratt as 'the people and organisations that connect around a shared purpose' (Pratt et al., 2005). The cardiovascular system, lungs and the rest of the body are a whole system with the shared purpose of keeping someone alive. A *complex adaptive system* has been described by Stacey to describe the ongoing creative interactions between different factors and systems (Stacey, 1996) – the changes in a body as it ages demonstrate how various bodily functions adapt and change in concert.

Hard, soft and complex adaptive systems help to see different aspects of a whole system. Each looks at a different aspect of connections. Senge (1993) describes systems thinking as the 'fifth discipline' of a learning organisation, 'the discipline to connect the other disciplines'. This may be the most important message from this chapter – everything connects in one way or another and you are more likely to do good if you consider in every situation which connections matter. Capra has written a series of books about connections; if you want to know more about systems theory try his book *The Web of Life* (Capra, 1997).

Capra (1997) points out that we in the West devalue connections compared with the East. This is certainly true in medicine where the prime aim is the diagnosis of discrete diseases. Systems thinking is perhaps more difficult for those of us who have come through medical education. By comparison, many nurses have been particularly concerned with family and community relationships, so the central importance of connections may be quite obvious to you. If this chapter seems to be stating the glaringly obvious, be reassured – it is. You already know this. But you will need to act systematically on this knowledge and that is not always easy.

Something that confronts all of us when systematically relying on systems is that we must in part let go of our previous habit of direct personal control. This may give you an uncomfortable feeling that everything is out of control. Indeed, there are quite likely to be some links in the chain that are not strong enough. When working with system ideas you face two challenges – to be reassured that the systems you are describing are good (they really must allow connections) and managing your own anxieties when learning to trust them. It takes patience.

Ways in which systems thinking can help you practically

System mapping can help you to see the practical value of systems thinking. Merely writing on a large piece of paper the range of factors relevant to your concern can show the multiple connections in seemingly simple situations. For example, knowing the array of educational courses or self-help groups can give you a sense that you know the options. You can help a patient to see the multiple interconnections in their own body by a drawing that displays how various things connect.

Recognising nodes in a system helps you to plan a set of services. Nodes are places where different systems connect. At nodes, participants learn about each, gaining windows into quite different worlds of understanding. They are the means of connecting networks of networks. Consider a railway network. Each line has its own stations and trains. But at some stations you can get onto another line which connects with a completely different set of stations. This is a node. Examples of nodes are away days, coffee breaks, social occasions, cross-portfolio meetings, cross-organisational planning groups, conferences, and international partnerships for research. In each of these, the potential exists for exploring diverse things that interest you.

Nodes offer particular opportunities for sharing and accessing knowledge, building cross-organisational relationships and getting a better sense of the whole healthcare endeavour. They need to be facilitated as learning spaces where participants enjoy learning from and with each other. Here they can meet others, exchange views, form alliances and create projects together. When these are comfortable, reflective and welcoming places they encourage this. When they feel unfriendly and blaming they produce a stifling atmosphere that inhibits creative interaction.

Practice of whole systems thinking

This section includes exercises to help you to be skilled at the four key areas:

1. identify the breadth of issues involved (rapid appraisal)
2. hold the story (cycles of inquiry)
3. plan coordinated changes (backwards mapping)
4. maintain personal balance.

Identify the breadth of issues involved (rapid appraisal)

General principles when appraising situations quickly
To get a good start in a new situation you need to understand it quickly. One technique that can help is *rapid appraisal*. It requires an understanding of the

story so far from different perspectives. It uses *written literature, personal observations* and *interviews of key informants*. Your appraisal should help you to make interpretations you had not considered at the outset, as well as allowing you to record your first impressions and gut instincts. You should:

- Describe the various individual and shared stories and the social forces that shape them.
- Identify who attends what meetings and what projects and policies are developed through them.
- Reveal various subgroups and shadow groups, alliances and networks that administer authority and power.
- Reveal what vision the stakeholders say they have and the extent to which their actions are true to that vision.
- Anticipate future surprises.

Implications for the clinical encounter
You can ask patients general and specific questions about their past and future, to see more of the person beyond their diagnoses.

Implications for managing case loads and influencing decision making
Rapid appraisal can be used to identify which groups of people need to be part of your project team and whose support you need to ensure a successful outcome.

Implications for yourself
Rapid appraisal techniques will help you to quickly get the measure of new situations in both your personal and professional lives.

Exercise: devise a rapid appraisal
Consider your management of a dying patient. Brainstorm a list of people who you may need to involve. Make sure that this includes people outside your immediate field of view but relevant to a good outcome. To quickly understand the breadth of people consider: what literature will you read and why?, who from your stakeholder list will you interview and what questions will you ask?, what situations will you observe and for what will you be looking? Then do it. Write down your new understanding of the situation.

Reflect on what new insights your rapid appraisal has given you about an effective approach. In particular:

- Have you recognised the web of relationships that will affect how things go?
- Does your plan bring relevant stakeholders into the conversation? Does it include the creation of learning spaces where people of

different backgrounds can consider the implications of different courses of action and then transfer this learning to other places? Have you identified how these spaces can best be facilitated?

- Have you identified a need for high performance multidisciplinary teams and have you plans to build them?
- What are you going to do about your own need for personal balance?

Hold the story (cycles of inquiry)

General principles when bringing a whole story into view

We describe ourselves to others through stories. The desire to describe a coherent life story is a major motivator. So we present our story in ways that feel right at the time, depending on who we are talking to and what we want to achieve. Improving the health of someone means getting beyond these immediate interpretations. By giving people the space to say more fully what has happened in the past and the impact it had on them and what they would really like to happen in the future, we can better identify what health means to someone at this stage of their life and what future plans would be the best ones to make.

We can discern a fuller, more truthful and meaningful life story by separating reflections on the past from explorations of future possibilities and that again from practical plans. This separation helps to avoid subconscious manipulation of the story to achieve something that has only transient importance. For example, a discussion of preferred place of burial may be completely prevented by a patient's concern about the cost and incon-venience to others of certain options. By first exploring past meanings and various future options, planning can better consider a variety of considera-tions and consequently arrive at the best compromise.

Implications for the clinical encounter

You can encourage patients to undertake their own inquiries about their own health. For example by keeping a diary of symptoms, exploring self-help opportunities through the internet, or experimenting with different treatments.

Implications for managing case loads and influencing decision making

Cycles of enquiry enable you to reflect systematically and develop a culture of continuous improvement within your team. This is particularly important if, as a team leader, you are building a learning organisation (see Chapter 8).

Implications for yourself

You too need to be skilled at rigorous inquiries and use these to learn.

Exercise: devise three cycles of inquiry

Agree with your planning team, or with a patient, to undergo three connected discussions about something of importance. The first is concerned with *establishing what it is* (perhaps their existing plans or a service configuration); the second gains *insights into new ways of doing things*; the third explores how those insights help to *plan useful changes*.

For each stage, or cycle, look at whatever data you have (e.g. existing plans) to move the discussion from abstract ideas to concrete plans. In a service development initiative, a pilot project is a helpful way to see what it might look like. During the second stage, you should consider all ideas, without immediately finding reasons why they are impractical – this helps to open the mind to new possibilities. If people have had a chance to mull over these new ideas for a while before the final stage of making new plans, they may come to see their advantages and disadvantages better.

Plan coordinated changes (backwards mapping)

General principles when using backwards mapping

You are probably familiar with the technique of forcefield analysis to analyse obstacles and enablers to coordinated change at one point. Backwards mapping is a technique that allows various obstacles and enablers at various points. Backwards mapping starts with a clear description of what is wanted at the most peripheral or distant point in the organisation. You then work backwards from this to identify what is needed at various stages beforehand. It helps you to see things from other people's points of view. This produces a plan that can be visualised on a timeline. Doing the exercise well gives you confidence that the timeline will bring everything together at the right time.

This approach quickly demonstrates that many things need to come together at the same time and in the same place. These may come from different places – perhaps different disciplines, different parts of a building or from different organisations. For example, if you want receptionists to provide reliable information about the organisation, they need to know staff movements. One step back from this you need all staff to provide up-to-date information about their movements.

Backwards mapping helps not only to achieve a certain goal. It also helps you to identify a set of places at which different paths can usefully cross. These are the nodes we mentioned earlier in the chapter. By standing back and considering the potential value of a node, you may find other things that can usefully come together there – for example, you may recognise that the person who holds the list of people's availabilities should also hold the timetable of meetings, annual leave and social events.

When you are aware of the various domains that may matter to you to keep these paths crossing efficiently, you can start building a multipurpose database that will quickly help you to access the people you need when you need to. Backwards mapping can also help you to cascade information through nodes. Getting the order of cascade right is important if those charged with minding a node are to amalgamate data in time to help the team to make decisions. This can be helpful when, as a leader of service change, you want to keep your constituents informed.

The same principle of working backwards can help produce personal career and learning plans. They help to plan educational events and manage projects. In each case you:

1   Identify what needs to happen and when.
2   Deduce what needs to be in place one step before this.
3   Identify the various things needed to bring this about and so on.

Use a big piece of paper and leave it on the wall, to become familiar with all the connections.

Implications for the clinical encounter
You can help a patient to plan improvement of their own health by mapping backwards from various goals, identifying a set of prior steps.

Implications for managing case loads and influencing decision making
You can use backwards mapping and sets of coordinated timelines to show when information needs to be transferred from one team to another. It displays to everyone how different activities are relevant to each other and to the management of the patient pathway.

Implications for yourself
The backwards mapping technique helps to plan any situation, from a dinner party to long-term career plans. It will help you to effectively juggle different portfolios.

Exercise: draw a backwards map
Decide a future event of importance – perhaps the death of a patient or the stage where they lose certain abilities. Identify different factors and people that will matter at that time. Write down what you want to happen between them (e.g. communication, support, knowledge).

Complete a backwards map. On a large piece of paper, write down what you need to achieve one step back for each of these factors/people. Then work backwards again to reveal the sequence of things that need to happen from now onwards. Stand back and see if it makes sense. Rewrite it as a timeline of tasks.

Maintain personal balance

General principles about balance, personally and professionally

Being balanced requires a degree of strength in all dimensions of health – physical, mental, social and spiritual. You may find it helpful at pivotal moments in your life to reflect on what you need in each of these domains for the challenges ahead and devise a plan to achieve them. Health can be improved by doing everyday things differently. You can take the stairs rather than a lift, centre yourself in between appointments and use images and breathing to calm inner voices of doubt. You can train all your senses to be alert in the moment.

Techniques that help you to be alive in the moment can be found in the literature of stress management, career and life management, self-development, spirituality and meditation. Different people prefer a different combination of approaches.

Things you can do to remain buoyant in the moment include the following:

- Use images and phrases that keep you alive in the present. With the best will in the world, the pressures of daily life will at times force you to feel that you have 'lost the plot'. This can be a prolonged 'dark night of the soul' or a temporary distraction. It can even be your dominant habit. You can reduce the damaging effects of this by using images and phrases that remind you of times when you could see things in a more optimistic way. The aim is to keep you balanced and alive.
- A common threat to balance is when engaging with those who see things differently from you, especially when they are critical of you. In these situations, it may help to remind yourself that you can learn from them. It may be better to understand and help them than to assert your authority or prove them wrong. You should anticipate these moments of misunderstanding and have to hand the evidence to set right incorrect facts.
- You may need to rise above the stress of the moment that will lead you to say or do things you will regret. Images that are meaningful to you may help you to keep alive in the present. From your past you may find helpful pictures, completed work, or friends. From your future you may find useful the plans that remind you of your intended trajectory. Your aim is to keep focused on what the people around you are saying, both in words and what they really mean. You need to keep at bay the internal voices that cause self-doubt. You need to be able to feel the tensions around you and inside you and rise above these to reach out to understand the others.

- In the chapter on transformational leadership (Chapter 8) we will introduce you the techniques of visualisation and role play to help you remain balanced in complex situations.
- A simple rule is an easy-to-remember directive that can switch on a mental model. 'Fight to the death' is a simple rule that relates to the mental model of 'I will overcome my adversaries'. 'The customer is always right' is a simple rule that relates to the mental model of 'the best way to gain customers is to keep them happy'. It is time well spent to examine what mental models you want and what simple rules will switch them on.

Implications for the clinical encounter
Patients commonly feel lost and isolated. You can help them to find images and words that keep them going while they grope for coherence.

Implications for managing case loads and influencing decision making
Policy must help staff to manage stress and remain alert in the midst of change and conflict. Team leader support and good team working are essential to develop mutually affirming images.

Implications for yourself
You will need to discover those images and phrases that keep you alive in the moment. You will need to practise them and be reflective about the effect they have on you. If you are unable to be alive, happy and effective in the middle of the multiple forces that threaten to knock you off balance, you may need to reconsider your plan.

Exercise: devise a plan for personal balance
Brainstorm the things you need for yourself when supporting a patient, family and team through a terminal illness.

Draw on a piece of paper a set of 'boats' and attach a label to each that summarises a key theme from this brainstorm – things that are important to you. Continue until you can think of no more areas/boats. Look at each in turn and score each from −5 to +5; that is, your satisfaction with the present situation. In red pen, draw lines to connect those 'boats' that are so closely connected they strongly need one another for either to be aide to move forward.

Redraw the whole picture on a grid marked −5 to +5, rearranging the boats on the appropriate grid marking and put those with red pen together. Stand back and look at the overall pattern seeking ways to move forward those 'boats' that are behind and also discerning things that are not even on the paper that might help to produce a better overall pattern.

In another colour pen (say, green) test new ideas – draw new boats that may help move the others forwards. Write notes to yourself about what you are learning about yourself. Remember, this is for your eyes only. Be prepared to put things on that you had previously thought to be unthinkable – they may provide clues to your best strategy.

Also in green indicate boats you intend to move forward and backwards in the next period. Write conclusions for action. Write the date on the picture and keep it safe so you can review it another time.

Summary

We have used a particularly challenging and complex situation – managing death – to illustrate how whole systems thinking can help you improve care for patients and lead service development. In the next chapter, you will learn more about what it means to coordinate change throughout a whole system and to bring along with you the constituencies for whom you are a leader.

References

Capra, F. (1997) *The Web of Life*. London, Flamingo.
Checkland, P. (1995) *Systems Thinking, Systems Practice*. Bath, Wiley.
Pratt, J., Gordon, P. and Plamping, D. (2005) *Working Whole Systems: putting theory into practice in organisations*, 2nd edn. Oxford, Radcliffe Publishing.
Senge, P. (1993) *The Fifth Discipline*. London, Century Hutchinson.
Stacey, R. (1996) *Complexity and Creativity in Organisations*. San Francisco, Berrett-Koehler.
Thomas, P. (2006) *Integrating Primary Health Care – leading, managing, facilitating*. Oxford, Radcliffe Publishing.

8   Transformational leadership

Deirdre Kelley-Patterson and Paul Thomas

Introduction

Leadership or transformation is concerned with coordinated change throughout the whole system. As an advanced practitioner you need to be such a leader when you help a patient to transform their understanding of their future in the light of their illnesses; and also as a leader of service developments when you help team members to see why improvement or innovation is needed.

In our previous chapter on whole systems thinking, we introduced you to four stages in a transformational process:

1   identify the breadth of issues involved
2   hold the story
3   plan coordinated changes
4   maintain personal balance.

You may like to reread this section, because in this chapter, we build from it to reveal ways for you to lead each of these stages.

Several aspects of this chapter are adapted from Thomas (2006).

Before you begin reading, consider *Case study 8.1*.

Case study 8.1 Leadership style

A community matron contemplates how she can transform practice to support patients who wish to die at home, in an environment where admittance to hospital is regarded as normal practice. As she reflects on a change strategy, she recognises that the individuals supporting patients and their families differ in terms of experience, self-confidence and professional background. Confident team members, with experience of acting as a patient advocate, will need her to enable and facilitate, but might feel frustrated and undermined if she behaved in a highly directive way. Less experienced and confident members could not be left without direction and might at times require her active intervention. Not only will she need to be sensitive to the wishes of the patient and his family but also to the differing needs of the team and the challenges of the dominant culture. As these three elements shift and change, so she will need to vary her leadership style and demonstrate behavioural flexibility. No one best way of leading will suit all situations.

Leadership – heroic or transformational?

The image we so often have of a leader is that of a heroic, pioneering cowboy carving a lonely path through uncharted territory. Leaders of transformation cannot be such loners because the job is to help others to do things for themselves. These leaders are 'sense makers', helping people to see the sense of doing things in a coordinated way. Transformational leaders must get under the skin of those they serve and empower all involved to think for themselves, interact and together find ways to connect their personal insights to see a bigger picture.

While the role of the advanced primary care practitioner, as envisioned in the NHS Improvement Plan (Department of Health, 2004), is largely sketched in clinical terms, there is both a 'change agent' and empowerment tone to much of the role description. Advanced practitioners in primary care are employed to 'teach and educate', be 'highly visible and in charge of care', 'be seen by colleagues across agencies as having the key role'.

In this chapter, you will be introduced to some of the key approaches to leadership that have helped to shape our expectations of how a leader should behave. In particular, we argue that leadership, in the context of the advanced practitioner role, is about helping to create a learning environment where people are supported to take calculated risks in complex and uncertain situations. To be effective you have to see the world of primary care as a system, make sense of your role in this system and support others to learn by acting as steward, teacher and systems guide.

For example, one of the identified competences for community matrons and case managers in primary care is to 'enable individuals with long-term conditions to manage their medicines' (DH, 2005). Clearly an approach that relies on patient education is important but not sufficient to meet this competence unit. Rather, to be effective, you will have to consider your patient's physical and mental capabilities, their attitude and levels of motivation, the role of carers and family and possibly even the services and support offered by the local pharmacy. Any attempt to address this need, which focuses on only one of these dimensions, is likely to be less than adequate. Effective service leadership depends not only on your understanding and ability to influence change in a complex situation, but also on your ability to help a large number of other people to understand this bigger picture so that they start to think and behave differently.

At the end of the chapter we include some techniques and exercises to help you develop your leadership skills in the context of whole systems thinking.

Leadership – many approaches: multiple demands

Type 'leadership' into an internet search engine and you will pull up around 150,000,000 references. These will point you towards numerous academic journals, self-improvement programmes, consultancy services, dictionaries and encyclopaedias offering a plethora of (slightly) differing definitions. Within a few minutes you will begin to appreciate that these resources generate more questions than they answer. Questions such as:

- Do personal qualities matter?
- What is the difference between a manager and a leader?
- Can I be trained to be an effective leader?
- Can we change our ways of behaving?
- What behaviours are most effective in which contexts?

To help simplify the territory we use a simple framework to help us understand the many approaches to leadership and, more importantly, to understand what leadership means in a complex primary care setting (see Figure 8.1).

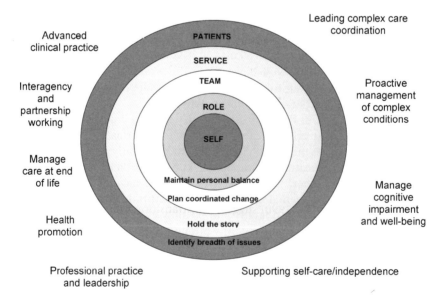

Figure 8.1 Advanced practitioner leadership framework

This model positions the advanced practitioner in the centre of a system that requires competence in a complex network of interrelated behaviours. Not only must the practitioner master these competences so as to provide a patient-centred service but s/he must:

- **maintain personal balance** by understanding what personal qualities are brought to the situation and developing emotional resilience so as to remain buoyant as s/he rides the waves of changes and manages challenges
- **plan coordinated change** through other people and bring diverse people together as members of a high-performance team
- **hold the story** by maintaining a complex network of *relationships* with colleagues and other stakeholders so as to continuously improve services
- **identify the breadth of issues involved** so as to generate a coherent vision of care for your patient and team.

Up until the 1960s, leadership was defined as a process of influencing or persuading people to do something (usually to achieve a specified goal). By the late 1980s, however, a paradigm shift was taking place and writers started to view leadership as a process of shaping meaning and developing 'learning' cultures which supported experimentation and empowered team members to solve problems in a systemic way.

Personal qualities and characteristics of leaders

One of the first questions you may have asked yourself when promoted into your current role is: 'Can I do this!', 'Have I got what it takes?' We all hold an image of what a 'good leader' looks like and are frequently anxious as to whether we measure up do this ideal. The NHS leadership qualities framework identifies five important personal qualities of effective leaders: self-belief, self-awareness, self-management, drive for improvement and personal integrity, a far cry from the popular pioneering cowboy image we referred to at the start of the chapter (NHS Institute for Innovation and Improvement, 2003).

Tichy and Devanna (1990) suggest that transformational leaders share a number of personal qualities:

- They see themselves as change agents and their own self-image (personal and professional) is that of someone who wants to make a difference and transform the organisation for which they are responsible.

- They are regarded by colleagues as courageous people who take a stand and are prepared to take prudent risks.
- They are people oriented, prepared to put trust in others, emotionally intelligent and committed to the empowerment of others.
- They hold firm to a set of core values which they are able to explain to others. They behave in ways that are congruent with their value positions.
- They are lifelong learners, able to talk about mistakes they have made and to view mistakes as learning opportunities.
- They have the ability to deal with complexity, ambiguity and uncertainty. They can frame problems in a complex, changing world and see the big picture.
- They are visionaries with the ability to dream, the ability to translate those dreams and images so that other people can share them.

These qualities differentiate the transformational leader from the transactional – a leader who is good at dealing with the everyday demands of a stable and predictable world. You might think of this as the difference between a leader and an effective manager. As an advanced practitioner, you may not possess all these qualities (they are, after all, based on CEOs of multinational corporations and not newly promoted professionals in a PCT!) but you can probably recognise at least some of these in colleagues and managers.

Relationships and the leader style and behaviour

The chances are that, at some stage of your journey from a newly qualified professional to an advanced practitioner with management responsibility, you have been offered training in areas such as performance management, conflict resolution or influencing skills. Unpinning courses of this kind is the assumption that leadership is a skill rather than a quality, something that can be learnt rather than something you 'just have'. You may have asked yourself even if I'm not a 'natural' leader can I be trained up?

When considering the way in which you respond to different stakeholders or behave with different team members you will appreciate that we modify our style to suit the situation. Leadership-style training and behaviour modification strategies were a popular focus of writing in the 1960s. Much of the research at that time was aimed at identifying the component elements of different leadership styles and attempting to identify which styles were most effective. For example, researchers at Ohio State University (Fleishman, 1953) identified two generic styles of leadership which they labelled 'initiating structure styles' (concerned with managing tasks) and 'consideration styles' (concerned with subordinates' needs and expectations). Today we expect leaders to demonstrate that they can confidently deal with both the technical or operational aspects of the role as well as manage people.

In our medicines management scenario, there are a number of planning, organising and controlling challenges (what quantity of medication should be kept by the patient, how will the medication be delivered to the patient, in what form/types of container, who will monitor patient compliance etc.) as well as human ones (dealing with resistance, allaying fears, motivating several stakeholders to engage with and continue to work with the new system). You will have to develop the skills and knowledge to manage both types of challenge when changing this system and you will need the mental flexibility and sensitivity to assess when to be concerned with the practical and mechanical and when to deal with the emotional.

Responding to the demands of the service: the importance of the situation

By the 1970s writers on leadership (see, for example, Fiedler, 1967; Adair, 1979) were arguing for a 'contingency' approach – the idea that leaders need to adapt their behaviour and style to the demands of the situation they encounter. Consider the community matron competency – *develop, sustain and evaluate collaborative work with others*. When working closely with other professionals there are many factors in the situation that you might 'read' before deciding how to act. How specific is the task or project that you have to achieve, what is the timescale, how experienced are other team members, have you worked with them before? Successful leaders are able to adapt their behaviour to meet the needs of the situation.

It may sometimes be appropriate to issue instructions and performance manage (initiating structure); on other occasions consultation and delegation (consideration) will be far more effective.

Leadership, patient-centred approaches

From the studies referred to earlier, we can conclude that effective leaders:

- have self-knowledge and are aware of their personal strengths and weaknesses; in particular, the transformational leader has vision, engages with change, empowers others and has high emotional intelligence
- are capable of modifying their personal style so as to set direction for and motivate a team

- are sensitive to the demands of the situation, flexible in responding to different priorities and capable of delivering a service through other people.

Bryman (1999) argues that the common theme uniting all these approaches is that leadership is primarily a task of influencing a group of followers to achieve goals. When we think about this from the perspective of primary care it raises a number of problems:

- The concept of 'followership' sits uneasily when dealing with patients, carers, peers and colleagues from multidisciplinary backgrounds. In the context of your role as an advanced practitioner, it is likely that many decisions are taken by members of a team not an individual leader. Professionals often share leadership (Yukl, 1998) depending on the nature of the issue or condition; the mantle of leader is passed to the professional best placed to offer expert advice at that point in time. In terms of the leadership in healthcare, it may be more helpful to think in terms of networks of leaders (Thomas, 2006).
- There is a tendency in some of the earlier writing on leadership to ignore issues of power and culture – to see leadership as a process of making a rational choice of a behaviour that will 'fit' the assessed demands of the situation. The reality of the many situations is that our choice of options is constrained by policy, professional boundaries or patient choice. Compromises have to be struck, full participation, not just consultation, is needed frequently, and decision-making partnerships have to be created.

So we need a new way of thinking about leadership – a framework to help us to think through the complexities of transforming primary care practice. Alan Bryman (1999: 30) describes this new way of thinking as the 'management of meaning'. Here the leader is someone who 'defines organisational reality through the articulation of a vision, mission and values'. In this new paradigm of leadership, the advanced practitioner must legitimise his/her position and contribution through an ability to shape others' understanding of the vision.

S/he can't rely on expertise or professional status to influence a situation but must rather use explanation and empowerment to help others make informed choices. This is particularly important, as new policy developments in health and social care require a new kind of leadership that enables collaboration across boundaries. Multiagency working models of transformational leadership stress the importance of skills such as having a vision and facilitating a strategic direction across organisations.

Similarly, Weick (1995) sees the leader as a 'sense maker' whose role is not to help groups achieve goals but to trust that people will change when meaning and relevance are clear: a shift from leading to empowering. Empowerment means helping patients, carers and colleagues to understand that there are no certain outcomes and that obstacles and challenges are not predictable. Leadership as 'sense making' helps people to learn from others and harmonise their efforts. It helps people to become confident in their skills as listeners and as reflective practitioners. It is concerned with long-term as well as short-term goals. For the long term, you must build your own infra-structure of personal support, competent teams, sources of reliable informa-tion and time for yourself. Alimo-Metcalfe and Alban-Metcalfe (2000: 27) conclude that 'transactional competencies of management, while crucial, are simply not sufficient on their own', but that leadership in healthcare should be 'fundamentally about engaging others as partners in developing and achieving the shared vision'. They term this 'connectedness'.

One of the most important contributions of the new paradigm is that it extends our understanding of transformational leadership to take into account the leader's work in generating organisational learning and innova-tion. Transformational leaders help others to look for and make sense of the 'new' and to construct their own innovative approaches for engaging with this new way of looking at the world.

Creating a culture which fosters learning and innovation requires attention to five key activities with which leaders must engage:

1   systematic problem solving – scientific approaches not guesswork, data not assumptions
2   ongoing experimentation – both small-scale and larger 'demonstra-tion projects'
3   learning from past experience – systematic and open review to avoid constantly repeating past poor performance
4   learning from others – 'enthusiastic borrowing' replacing the 'not-invented-here' syndrome
5   transferring knowledge quickly and efficiently through the organi-sation/between organisations (Garvin, 1993)

> The new view of leadership in learning organizations centres on subtler and more important tasks. In a learning organization, leaders are designers, stewards, and teachers. They are responsible for building organizations where people continually expand their cap-abilities to understand complexity, clarify vision, and improve shared mental models – that is, they are responsible for learning.
>
> (Senge, 1990: 7)

Implications for advanced practitioners

From all this writing and research we suggest that there are a number of simple rules of thumb for effective leadership:

1 **Identify the breadth of issues involved**. Leaders have to keep the big picture firmly in mind and help other team members visualise patterns and outcomes. By connecting a complex set of parameters, you help multiple stakeholders understand the effect of their individual action on whole systems change. Help others participate and appraise the forces for change and the breadth of issues involved.

2 **Hold the story**. Leaders are a point of connection – they help others to understand the past and plan the future. In a complex situation, they help to unravel mess and focus on what is important. As a leader you can help to create and sustain nodes where systems connect (see Chapter 7).

3 **Plan coordinated changes**. When planning future care for a patient several things will need to change at the same time. Building a high-performance team, capable of learning from experience and tackling new challenges in an innovative and creative way, is the key here.

4 **Maintain personal balance**. Thinking at so many different levels and appreciating the contributions of so many different people can leave you unsure about who you are – you can feel torn in many directions. Leaders are emotionally resilient.

In the following section, we include a series of exercises to help you with these simple rules.

Strategies and techniques for enhancing effectiveness

Identify the breadth of issues

Whole system change needs people from throughout the system to be mindful of the effect their actions have on others. When you understand what it is like from someone else's perspective you become better able to adapt your own behaviour to be complementary to theirs. This empathy allows you to feel on the same side rather than an adversary, helps to build trusted relationships and promotes team working.

In the previous chapter, we explained how you could use three cycles of inquiry to reveal a fuller, more reliable and enduring story than the version that is most convenient at the time. You can do this with a patient or with large numbers of people. To do this well it helps to see things through the eyes of that person/people. You can practise this through visualisation or role play.

Visualisation is a process where you step back from the noise and pressures of the everyday, let your mind freewheel and mentally role play situations. Find a quiet place where you will not be disturbed and make yourself comfortable. First, quickly imagine in as much detail as you can what it is you hope to achieve. Then put this out of your mind (don't worry, it will come back later and in a more coherent form). Use any relaxation technique with which you are familiar and comfortable (you need to ensure that you clear your mind of the pressures of the moment). Now that you are in a peaceful place (mentally) you are ready to start the visualisation.

Search your mind's eye for the person/people/situation you are concerned about. When you find them first look at the surroundings – where are you? Is it a room? What can you see in it? Then let the scenario unfold. First, feel your way into the other person/people. What is their interest in this? What other related concerns do they have? What approach from you will appeal to them?

Then focus on yourself. Engage with the individuals or groups. Remove from what you intended to say the things that will turn them away. Be reasonable, balanced and invincible. Watch yourself achieve the things you want and provide the information they want. Watch them agree. Note where they do not. When you are finished allow yourself to come back to the room. Write down what you have learned.

Hold the story

Leaders are vital points of connection – the junction in a network of activity and information. By building the capability of the network you help to create learning organisations.

A learning network is characterised by interactions with a wide range of people. Some of these people may belong to the primary care team, others may meet to undertake particular tasks as part of a multiagency project. So people may come and go throughout a working cycle. This is important where people are employed in different shifts and duties as currently happens in residential work. A network can accommodate a much wider range of values and individual professional approaches to the task than a team. It follows, therefore, that there can be agreement only on the most overall and generalised goals and values and within this framework some highly individualistic approaches to practice may be tolerated and respected. There are many networks throughout the NHS. Find out what is available and try to join one.

Plan coordinated changes

The important message here is to remember that in this chapter we are focusing on transformational leadership – and not on planning as a solitary or isolated activity. Think about how you can build a high-performing team (which includes professional colleagues, carers and the patient). These teams must be empowered to take responsibility for the success of the change. The teams need to reflect as far as possible the diversity of perspectives from the whole system you are working with, even bits of it that seem alarming and alien. Different team members can therefore provide insight into how different constituencies think and feel in response to a change initiative (this will feel uncomfortable at times – it is much easier to invite people with whom you get on and who 'see things your way').

Regular communication with your team is essential; this keeps everyone motivated to achieve your shared goals. Action plans need to be negotiated, documented and later checked for completion; this gives confidence in progress and in each other's skills. Protected time is needed for face-to-face meetings to revisit shared vision and to identify new problems and new possibilities. This helps to keep the whole group together and airs disagreements in private. Remember to demonstrate that you appreciate both the contribution of team members but also their anxiety and frustration at times of challenge or uncertainty. Appreciation demonstrates that you recognise how frightened people can be when out of their comfort zones. This makes them less able to learn and do what most needs to be done.

You can empower people to look at these difficult things by helping them to put temporary boundaries around situations that enable them to work through realistic but ambitious plans. You can do this by seeing change as 'incremental revolution' (Thomas, 2006).

Maintain personal balance

From Chapter 7, you will appreciate that being balanced requires a degree of strength in all dimensions of health – physical, mental, social and spiritual. You may find it helpful at pivotal moments in your life to reflect on what you need in each of these domains for the challenges ahead and devise a plan to achieve them.

Techniques that may help to keep you focused on your own health include personal development planning, 360° appraisal and developing emotional resilience. The emotionally resilient practitioner is able to recover quickly from illness, change or misfortune and can remain buoyant as s/he rides the waves of change and turbulence. Emotionally resilient people understand that they have to look for the positive in difficult situations – they see difficulties and challenges as learning opportunities. Deliberately and systematically looking for the positive in a situation will help you build a range of strategies to help you cope. Don't try to do everything at once. Your plan might identify three areas where you need to improve your resilience skills, but that doesn't mean you should try to accomplish them all at once. Instead, select one area that is the most important to you to work on first. Plan several achievable and time-limited goals. Breaking your larger goals into small achievable bits is the best way to successfully complete the change process.

Look for small gains, minor successes, find opportunities for humour and fun, take a short break or some exercise and, most importantly, pursue novel and creative thoughts and actions – doing something new and different really will help. A blaming or dismissive mindset will not recognise the good that exists in difficult situations and will block imaginative thinking about ways forward. When something seems wrong it may well indicate that something needs to be done (it may not) – but it does not necessarily tell you what to do. Often something that seems to be wrong does not need to be removed, but complemented by other things. Often the thing that is obstructing progress is out of your immediate vision and you need to look more broadly – the problem may be you!

As a transformational leader, you have some responsibility for helping your team cope – to 'run with the ball' (Thomas, 2006). You can help team members develop emotional resilience by devising an atmosphere of trust and mutual understanding. This requires that all team members become prepared to give things a go and be unafraid to fall. They must know from experience that when they can't quite pull things off, the team will support them, laugh with them and help them to learn how to pull it off next time. Shared projects are a good way to learn and practise these team skills.

Summary

In this chapter, we worked with a definition of transformational change that prioritises the change agent and empowerment dimensions of leadership. The effective practitioner is someone who shapes a vision of a desired future and persuades others to move with them to that future. Leaders of transformation know that individual actions can have unpredictable effects (remember the chaos theory butterfly that flapped its wings and caused a hurricane on the other side of the world). As a transformational leader in primary care, you will not be able to control events, people or situations. However, you can, like the butterfly, have a powerful and significant impact on the whole system by acting as a guide, teacher and shaper.

References

Adair, J. (1979) *Action-centred Leadership*. Aldershot, Gower.

Alimo-Metcalfe, B. and Alban-Metcalfe, R. (2000) Heaven can wait. *Health Services Journal* 12 October, 26–29.

Bryman, A. (1999) Leadership in organisations. In Clegg, S., Hardy, C. and Nord, W. (eds) *Managing Organisations: current issues*. London, Sage.

Department of Health (DH) (2004) *The NHS Improvement Plan: putting people at the heart of public services*. London, HMSO.

Department of Health (DH) (2005) *Case Management Competencies Framework for the Care of People with Long-term Conditions*. London, DH.

Fiedler, F. E. (1967) *A Theory of Leadership Effectiveness*. New York, McGraw-Hill.

Fleishman E. A. (1953) The measurement of leadership attitudes in industry. *Journal of Applied Psychology* 38, 1, 153–158.

Garvin, D. A. (1993) Building a learning organisation. *Harvard Business Review* Jul/Aug 71, 4, 78–92

NHS Institute for Innovation and Improvement (2003) *The NHS Leadership Qualities Framework*. London, NHS Institute for Innovation and Improvement.

Senge, P. M. (1990) The leader's new work: building learning organizations. *Sloan Management Review* 32, 1, 7–23.

Thomas, P. (2006) *Integrating Primary Health Care – leading managing, facilitating*. Oxford, Radcliffe Publishing.

Tichy, N. M. and Devanna, M. A. (1990) *The Transformational Leader*. New York, Wiley.

Weick, K. E. (1995) *Sensemaking in Organizations*. California, Sage.

Yukl, G. (1998) *Leadership in Organizations*, 4th edn. Englewood Cliffs, NJ, Prentice-Hall.

9 Developing and sustaining the advanced practitioner role

Karen Elcock

Introduction

Evaluations of advanced roles have found that practitioners can feel isolated and unsupported (Castledine and Mason, 2003; Bryant-Lukosius et al., 2004). These feelings can lead to demotivation, frustration and job dissatisfaction. It is essential therefore that effective support mechanisms are in place if these roles are to be sustainable. This chapter focuses on three strategies that can help you to achieve this:

- mentorship
- action learning sets
- reflective practice.

In describing these strategies, the focus is on how you as a new or developing advanced practitioner can use them to help you develop in your role. This chapter will also be useful to those who have been asked to support colleagues in advanced practitioner roles.

Mentorship

Mentorship will be familiar to most nurses working in primary care as it is a requirement for all pre-registration and many post-registration nursing programmes. Mentorship in this context focuses on the support of students, with a particular emphasis on the assessment of the student's competence to practice (NMC, 2006). This chapter moves away from this prescriptive approach to one that is widely used in private organisations and is being increasingly adopted by the public sectors. Mentorship is seen as a strategy not only to support and equip staff with the skills they require to undertake their day-to-day role but also for developing staff to reach their potential (Cranwell-Ward et al., 2004) and a valuable recruitment and retention strategy (Clutterbuck, 2004).

What is mentoring?

There are a plethora of definitions for mentoring but the following is particularly relevant to those in advanced practitioner roles:

> Mentoring is a positive developmental activity. Mentors can discuss current issues relating to the mentee's work, offering insights into the ways the organisation works, how the informal networks operate and how they think about the challenges and opportunities they encounter.
>
> (Clutterbuck, 2004: 14)

This corresponds well with two of the core elements that McGee and Castledine (2003: 59) have identified as important if advanced practitioners are to fulfil the principal elements of their role, which are 'to challenge professional boundaries and pioneer innovations'. Understanding how organisations work is important to be able to influence change. Knowing what networks exist and how to access them is essential as they not only offer an additional source of advice and support but are also a resource for new ideas and ways of working.

Mentoring versus coaching

The terms mentoring and coaching are often seen as interchangeable but are very different approaches to developing staff. Coaching tends to focus on the development of specific skills and so the improvement of performance. The coach tends to be directive in their relationship, which is usually short term, until the required improvement in performance has been achieved. With mentoring the relationship focuses on the whole person and tends to be longer term in nature. These two approaches are not mutually exclusive; the neophyte advanced practitioner will need both approaches as they develop into their role and this mix of approaches is often called matrix mentoring, which is discussed later.

Why is mentoring important?

Mentorship and coaching are one of the underpinning principles of the education framework for community matrons and case managers (DH, 2006). Mentorship is seen as crucial not only to help inexperienced community matrons acquire new competencies but also as a strategy to support their professional development (DH, 2005) and develop as mentors themselves.

The NHS Leadership Centre (2004) identifies the benefits of an effective mentoring relationship as:

- improved understanding of work issues and exposure to different approaches to dealing with them
- a sounding board for ideas
- knowledge from someone in a similar role about the external environment and the characteristics and culture of the sector
- opportunities for self-learning
- a chance to focus on priorities
- an increase in confidence.

These benefits relate to both the mentee and the mentor, with mentors also gaining personal satisfaction from supporting and developing another.

Mentoring schemes

The traditional approach to mentoring is a one-to-one relationship between a mentor and mentee. While the mentor is usually senior to the mentee and is often seen as an expert this is not always necessary. Klasen and Clutterbuck (2002) and Cranwell-Ward et al. (2004) describe a number of other mentoring schemes, some of which are particularly applicable to the advanced practitioner in the community setting. These are:

- peer mentoring
- group mentoring
- across organisations (e.g. between different PCTs or NHS trusts)
- matrix mentoring.

Each of these approaches can be valuable, particularly when new roles are being established as there are often no or few experienced practitioners already in place to provide the mentorship required. See Table 9.1 for identifying which ones may suit you best.

Peer mentoring

Here two colleagues at the same or a similar level in an organisation agree to a mentoring relationship. With peer mentoring one person may agree to take on the role of mentor and one the role of the mentee or both may agree to take turns in the two roles. This relationship can work well as there is no hierarchical relationship which can be an obstructing factor in many mentoring relationships and is also valuable in reducing the isolation that individuals may feel in new roles. To get the most out of peer mentoring it is best to choose a mentor who has a different outlook or works in a different area to enable different perspectives to be shared. Choosing someone who is similar

Table 9.1 Choosing a mentorship scheme

	I am on a course	I am new to the role	I am established in my role
My role is unique or colleagues in similar roles are not easily accessible	• One to one • Matrix mentoring	• One to one • Across organisations mentoring • Matrix mentoring	• One to one • Across organisations mentoring
There are others in similar roles in my organisation	• One to one • Group mentoring • Matrix mentoring	• One to one • Peer mentoring • Group mentoring • Matrix mentoring	• One to one • Peer mentoring

to yourself or works closely with you is unlikely to offer you the opportunity to be challenged in your ideas and actions and so will fail to develop the skills and knowledge you seek.

Group mentoring

This approach uses one mentor to support a small group of mentees and is particularly useful in organisations where there are very few experienced staff to take on a mentor role. This format is usually set up by the employer or an educational establishment as part of a course and, consequently, you do not get to choose your mentor. This can be problematic if their mentorship style does not suit you or other members of the group. While it offers the support elements of a mentoring relationship, it is less likely to offer the personal development that you may seek, and is probably best used when a group of staff are new to a role within an organisation or undertaking a course together. A similar but less formal approach is team mentoring where a group of practitioners meet on a regular basis and support each other. Team mentoring is useful in an organisation where a number of new roles have been established at the same time and can help reduce isolation and offer opportunities to share and discuss the issues and problems that are arising from implementing the new role.

Across organisations

Identifying a mentor from another organisation should be considered when there is no one in your own organisation available or who can meet your needs or when you know of someone from another organisation who has a particular expertise that you feel you would benefit from. While this can take a little effort initially in setting up, it can be particularly valuable as the mentor can bring a fresh perspective to the issues that you bring to the meetings. Both organisations can benefit through the sharing of knowledge and experience and the mentee will often feel secure in this relationship as it is outside their own organisation. When seeking a mentor from another organisation, you need to have a clear idea of what you expect from the relationship and what you will require of the mentor in terms of time. An initial, informal meeting is helpful to clarify expectations on both sides before entering into a more formal arrangement.

Matrix mentoring

Matrix mentoring (see Table 9.2) is used when an individual needs access to a range of different skills and knowledge which one person is unlikely to be able to offer. This is particularly true when developing in a new role and/or undertaking a new course where a range of specific skills need to be developed. Although the term mentoring is used, in reality this is far more akin to coaching as the relationship will focus on specific skill development for a fixed period of time. Once the skill has been learnt the relationship will terminate (although maintaining contact is important as they become part of your informal network). Matrix mentoring often works alongside a more formal one-to-one relationship. The main mentor is important as they are the constant throughout this time and will help you identify the specific skills you need to develop and may be able to help suggest whom you can go to to learn these skills.

Table 9.2 Mentoring matrix

	Mentor			
	Coach A	**Coach B**	**Coach C**	**Coach D**
Skills to be learnt ↓	**GP**	**Clinical nurse, specialist palliative care**	**Clinical nurse specialist diabetes**	**Physiotherapist**
Skill A				X
Skill B	X			
Skill C			X	
Skill D		X		

Models of mentoring

A range of mentoring models exist from the structured to the unstructured and the formal to the informal (Klasen and Clutterbuck, 2002; Clutterbuck, 2004; Cranwell-Ward et al., 2004). Formal models tend to be implemented by the organisation or are a requirement of an academic course and the mentor is usually allocated to the mentee or the mentee is given a list of mentors from which to choose. Informal models are usually initiated by the mentee who perceives a need and seeks a mentor to help them achieve it. The need may be for personal or professional development or to meet a specific skill (and so more of a coaching relationship) or knowledge deficit.

Structured models will utilise an agreed format to the meetings, for example:

- an agenda or agreed content
- the frequency of the meetings
- whether to record any discussion that takes place
- expected outcomes or outputs from the meetings.

This approach may suit people who are new to mentoring as it gives structure to the meetings which can otherwise become rambling chats and lead to a sense of dissatisfaction for both parties. Unstructured models tend not to have an agreed format and can be perceived as more of a social event, the coming together and discussion which takes place being seen as important as any specific outcomes from the meetings. The unstructured format tends to works best where the mentor is experienced in mentoring or when the mentee is gaining confidence in their work role.

If you are undertaking a programme of study or just starting in a new post the formally structured model may be more helpful to you initially. You can then choose to move to one of the other less formal models depending on personal need, keeping the same mentor or a seeking a new one.

Choosing a mentor

Ideally, a mentor should not be someone who is in a line management position; neither do they necessarily have to be seen as an expert in your field of practice. Where possible you should choose the person you wish to be mentored by. In selecting the right mentor, you need to consider why you need a mentor at this moment in time and, therefore, what specific types of skill or knowledge they need to be able to offer you. It is also important to consider the additional qualities and skills you would expect them to have.

REFLECTION: Consider who in your past has been particularly effective in supporting you. What skills or qualities did they have that enabled this? Which of those skills and qualities do you possess?

Each person will seek a different set of skills and qualities in a mentor, but ones you may have considered important are:

- good communication skills
- good listening skills
- openness
- interested in the mentee
- knowledgeable
- approachable
- trustworthy
- ability to challenge
- supportive.

Developing the mentorship relationship

Having identified your mentor there are a number of steps that need to be taken before the relationship formally starts. It is useful to meet with your prospective mentor to clarify how the relationship will work. The first meeting should focus on getting to know each other, sharing information on previous posts held, past experiences, particular interests and areas of expertise are helpful but most important is the clarifying of expectations that you have of each other in the mentoring relationship. This first meeting can help to reassure both of you that the mentor can meet your needs and that an effective relationship can be built. Basic housekeeping also needs to be sorted, for example:

- Where will you meet?
- How long will you meet for?
- How often will you meet?
- Will an agenda be set and if so who by?
- What will you be expected to bring to each meeting?
- Will notes be taken at the meeting, by whom and kept by whom?

It helps to prepare for the first session by bringing with you:

- a reflective diary of recent activities/events that could be used as a starting point for discussion

- a specific problem or difficulty that is challenging you
- a personal SWOT analysis (see next point).

REFLECTION: Jot down what you think are:

- your current **s**trengths
- your current **w**eaknesses or areas that need developing
- **o**pportunities that exist to develop yourself and your role
- **t**hreats to you undertaking your role effectively.

Now consider which are the most important to you and which you wish to work on with your mentor.

What happens at the meetings?

The format of the meetings will have been agreed in advance but some structure is useful. A simple format is shown in Figure 9.1.

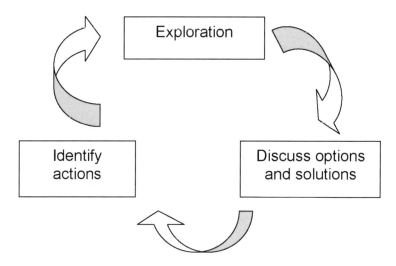

Figure 9.1 Format for mentoring meeting

Start with an exploration of the issue or challenge that you wish to work on to enable you to gain a better understanding of the problem. Consider the different options available to you and select the one(s) that you feel most comfortable with. Explore possible solutions to each option chosen and from these identify the actions that you are going to take. At the next meeting, you discuss the results from your actions and any issues that arose. If the issue you bring is quite complex, you may spend several sessions exploring and understanding the problem better, although it is always helpful to leave with some action points from each meeting even if they are not ones that will lead to an immediate solution.

Ending the mentoring relationship

Some mentoring relationships will come to a natural end either because all the expected outcomes have been achieved or because you have outgrown your mentor. In both cases, this is a positive outcome of the relationship. In other cases, the relationship fails due to people moving on, impacting work commitments or because the relationship itself isn't working for one or both parties involved. To prevent problems arising and to ensure that the relationship is continuing to meet its original objectives it is helpful to review progress at regular intervals. What has been achieved so far? What difficulties are arising and why? By reviewing progress you can then determine whether there is value in continuing the meetings and if not agree to end them in a way which will not leave either part feeling they have failed. Formal closure is important as it also offers each of you the opportunity to reflect on the experience and use the learning that arises from it in future mentoring relationships.

Have a look at *Case study 8.1* and reflect on any relevance it might have to your own situation.

Case study 9.1 Mentoring outside your organisation

Joan had recently been successful in applying for a post as a community matron. Hers was the first of these posts in her PCT and so there were no other community matrons who could mentor her. Feeling her line manager would be focused on her success (or lack of it) in this new role she decided to look outside the organisation for a mentor with whom she would feel safe to discuss her fears about undertaking this new post. Joan approached a lecturer she knew at the local university who had a community background and had supported her on a course in the past. After an initial discussion about Joan's expectations of the lecturer's role as a mentor they agreed to meet on a monthly basis with emails as an additional support mechanism. At their first meeting, two issues were identified. The first was managing the expectations of colleagues at work who were confused about her role, especially how it differed from their own and what she would or would not be doing in this new role. The second was the need to gain more experience in advanced assessment skills. They agreed the following action plan:

1   Joan would organise a meeting with colleagues at work to discuss her role and how they could work most effectively together.

2   Joan would keep a reflective diary of the interactions she had with colleagues at work that would be use at their monthly meetings to explore how she was managing their expectations and responses to her.

3   Joan should approach a GP to ask if he/she would act as a coach to enable her to develop her assessment skills.

Joan found using her diary enabled her to become far more objective about the way she responded to her colleagues. The meetings with her mentor allowed her to check out the appropriateness of her responses, to practise different approaches and agree new action plans where problems still existed. After six months Joan was feeling far more confident in her role and they decided to reduce the frequency of the meetings to four times a year with Joan using her reflective diary to record the events she wished to discuss when they met.

Action learning sets

Action learning has become popular within the health service as a strategy for leadership development (Thomas and Etheridge, 2004) and was used by the National Primary and Care Trust Development Programme (NATPACT) as the heart of its transformational change programme (NATPACT, 2005). Action learning sets are a way of promoting learning in the workplace, the word *action* being central to the success of the set, as learning occurs from the agreed actions that arise from the set meetings. While applicable to all levels of staff within an organisation, it can be particularly useful for people in new roles as it offers individuals dedicated personal time and space to explore work issues within a supportive framework at a stage in their career when they may still be trying to determine what their role is and how to enact it.

What is an action learning set?

An action learning set is a group of around five to eight people who meet on a regular basis to explore problems or challenges that an individual is facing in their work. Unlike team meetings where everyone talks and offers ideas, in learning sets the focus is always on the individual who is given dedicated time to talk about their own issue or problem which the set then works on with them (Weinstein, 1999). The set does not have to be made up from one professional group; in fact, having an interprofessional group can be far more rewarding as it allows different perspectives to be shared, can lead to a greater understanding of each other's roles and enable people to see the bigger picture.

There are essential elements that need to be in place if an action learning set is to be successful:

- Attendance is voluntary. All the members must want to participate and must commit to the meetings.
- The organisation must be willing to release staff to attend.
- Meetings need to take place on a regular and frequent basis (ideally every 4–6 weeks) to ensure that momentum is maintained and last for at least 2–3 hours.
- Ground rules must be agreed at the beginning and reinforced at each meeting.
- Having a skilled facilitator to ensure that the set keeps focused is helpful, however if one is not available don't let this stop you. If no one feels able to take on this role then it could be rotated through the group.

Common ground rules cover issues around:

- attendance
- timekeeping
- confidentiality
- acceptable behaviour amongst the group
- agreement on not giving advice.

REFLECTION: Consider which ones would be important to you and what you would expect under each of these headings.

Preparing for the set

Prior to the set meeting each member needs to identify an issue, challenge or opportunity they are facing at work or around their own professional development to bring with them to the meeting. It is important to choose something you have responsibility for, can influence or are personally involved in in some way, so that you can talk about it using 'I'. It must also be something that you do not have an answer for at this moment in time. Possible areas to consider are:

- communications with colleagues or others within or outside the organisation
- implementing a new system of care, e.g. for patient assessment
- responding to a new government initiative, e.g. part of a national service framework

- managing time
- managing complaints
- managing performance of others.

Before the first meeting you should ask yourself:

- What am I trying to do?
- What is preventing me from doing it?
- What might I be able to do about it?
- Who knows about the problem?
- Who cares about the problem?
- Who can do anything to help?

Starting the set

At each set meeting, revisit the ground rules. It is helpful to have them on a large sheet of paper which is put up on the wall to remind everyone what has been agreed and to refer to if the set moves away from the agreed rules. At the first meeting, you should also agree how the time will be allocated. Will you divide the time you have between each set member or give a longer amount of time to a small number of the set? A minimum of 30 minutes each is suggested with time also put aside for the beginning of the meeting where set members will feedback the results from their actions agreed at the last meeting and time at the end to briefly review how the set meeting has gone and what has been learnt. Where there is insufficient time for everyone to present, the facilitator can either identify if anyone has a particularly burning issue they wish to present or each member can give a two-minute presentation and the set members then agree who will present with a note taken of those who don't get the opportunity.

Some sets find it helpful to keep a brief record of what is explored and agreed at each meeting. This can be a useful aid to remind the set of what took place at the previous meeting and as a means of keeping track of what has been learnt over the period the set meetings are held. If you have a set facilitator then they can act as timekeeper, ensure you keep to the ground rules and act as scribe; if not, you may wish to appoint someone to take on this role at each set meeting.

Running the set

Each presenter has a maximum of 10 minutes to describe the issue they have brought to the meeting. The set members must listen and make no comments during this time. At the end of the presentation, each member has an opportunity to ask questions of the presenter to help clarify any areas which are unclear, challenge assumptions made and gain a clearer understanding of the issue. Most importantly, and probably the hardest part for the set members to remember, is not to give advice. Telling someone what you would do takes ownership away from the actions that arise, may not be the right advice for that person, reduces learning for both presenter and questioner or can lead to what Weinstein (1999) describes as 'verbal ping-pong' as the presenter responds with a series of 'yes but' and 'no because' responses which can prove frustrating for all involved. Through questioning the presenter is helped to gain new insights into the issue which leads them to identify potential actions or solutions which they agree with the group to try out. They then go away, try out the agreed actions and report back on the results at the next meeting. The report should describe what worked, what didn't work and ideas on why not. If the issue remains unresolved, the action learning cycle repeats resulting in a revised action plan to be implemented.

Both participation in the learning set and implementing the agreed action plan provide opportunities for learning which is achieved through reflection on the activities that took place.

Ending the set

Action learning sets should run for as long as the group members find them useful. One way of judging this is to make time at the end of each set meeting to reflect on what you gained by attending that day. If you find you are not gaining anything or if there are problems in the way the set is operating, then explore your concerns with the set, it could be the issue the set works on next time! Everyone's time is valuable so do not continue if nothing new is being gained. It is, however, valuable to formally close the set with a review of what has been achieved so that you end with a positive. It may also be appropriate to feedback the positives to your managers, thus keeping the door open for creating new action learning sets in the future.

Reflective practice

The ability to reflect on practice is an essential skill for the advanced practitioner (Hudson and Moore, 2006). It can be undertaken in isolation through the use of a reflective journal or be guided by a mentor or clinical supervisor (Johns, 1998). The reflective journal can also be a useful tool for guiding the meetings with a mentor, particularly when meetings do not occur very frequently or for identifying issues to present at action learning sets. There are a number of models or frameworks that can be used to structure your reflections and it is worth taking some time to look at these and determine which format suits you best (see Rolfe et al., 2001, for a useful review of the most popular models). Some are quite simple, others are more structured but each has basic elements in common: describing the incident, analysing what occurred, identifying learning and developing an action plan. Box 9.1 merges some of these ideas into a framework you could use.

Box 9.1 A framework for reflection

1   Describe the incident, issue or situation:

   • What happened or is not happening?
   • Who was involved?
   • How did you behave? How did others behave?
   • How did you and others feel about the situation?

2   Making sense of the experience:

   • What factors influenced your actions and the actions of others (consider your own level of knowledge and skills and your feelings about the situation and the people involved as well as other factors such as time, priorities and organisational politics)?

3   What have I learnt?

   • About myself – a knowledge or skills deficit or a particular expertise you hold
   • About others
   • About the organisation
   • How will this new knowledge influence me in the future?

4   Formulate an action plan:

   • What actions will you take to resolve the situation described?
   • What might the consequences of those actions be?

Keeping a reflective journal

An immediate response by most people is that they do not have time to keep a journal, but it does not have to take up much time and it is just like any other skill, something that becomes easier and quicker to complete the more you do it (see *Box 9.2*). If you are new to journaling it is useful to use a reflective model or framework to structure your thoughts; don't, however, feel constrained by the framework; if it doesn't quite fit your situation then modify it. As you become more experienced with reflecting, you will probably find that you no longer need it.

Box 9.2 Tips for keeping a reflective journal

- Use a loose-leaf folder or specific book to record your entries in
- If new to journaling, use a model/framework to structure your entries
- Pre-print/copy several copies of the model or framework with suitable gaps to fill in and put in your folder ready for use
- Have it to hand so you don't need to search for it
- Identify a time in your day/week when you will have space to complete it
- Aim to make a minimum of one entry every week
- If something happens at work that you think is important or affects you strongly, write down the key points and put the list in your journal until you have time to write it out in full
- Try to balance any 'negative entries' with positive ones

Deciding what to write is another challenge for many practitioners. It does not have to be a big event or necessarily something that went wrong. While it is always valuable to reflect on something that did not go well, it is also important to reflect on positive events. Why did something go well? What was it about yourself that made it a positive encounter? From reflecting on the positives, we can learn about our own strengths which is just as important as identifying our weaknesses. Often it is not a particular event that needs to be recorded but something more general or ongoing. For example, it may be around a particular relationship with a client or colleague or a particular organisational process that is frustrating you in some way. What is important is that you want to *write* about it. If it is significant to you then it is worth writing about.

Having completed a number of entries in your journal it is worthwhile taking time out to review them. Did you implement your action plans? Were they successful? If not what prevented their success? Are there any recurrent themes? What does this tell you about yourself? If you find recurrent themes in your journal or the inability to follow through on your actions take these to your next meeting with your mentor. Discussing them with another person may help you identify what is happening and why.

Lastly, remember that your journal is confidential; no one has the right to see what you have written.

Summary

The sense of isolation that many advanced practitioners feel can be managed through the proactive use of mentorship, action learning sets and reflection. Whether used alone or alongside each other they all require commitment in terms of time and energy to be successful. The benefits, however, are significant both personally and professionally and so well worth the investment.

References

Bryant-Lukosius, D., DiCenso, A., Browne, G. and Pinelli, J. (2004) Advanced practice nursing roles: development, implementation and evaluation. *Journal of Advanced Nursing* 48, 5, 519–529.

Castledine, G. and Mason, T. (2003) The development of a career pathway for advanced practitioners. In McGee, P. and Castledine, G. (eds) *Advanced Nursing Practice*, 2nd edn. Oxford, Blackwell Publishing.

Clutterbuck, D. (2004) *Everyone Needs a Mentor: fostering talents in your organisation*, 4th edn. London, Chartered Institute of Personnel Development.

Cranwell-Ward, J., Bossons, P. and Gover, S. (2004) *Mentoring: a Henley review of best practice*. Basingstoke, Palgrave Macmillan.

Department of Health (DH) (2005) *Supporting People with Long-term Conditions: liberating the talents of nurses who care for people with long-term conditions*. London, HMSO.

Department of Health (DH) (2006) *Caring for People with Long-term Conditions: an education framework for community matrons and case managers*. London, HMSO.

Hudson, A. J. and Moore, L. J. (2006) A new way of caring for older people in the community. *Nursing Standard* 20, 46, 41–47.

Johns, C. (1998) Knowing and realizing advanced practice though guided reflection. In Rolfe, G. and Fulbrook, P. (eds) *Advanced Nursing Practice*. Oxford, Butterworth Heineman.

Klasen, N. and Clutterbuck, D. (2002) *Implementing Mentoring Schemes: a practical guide to successful programmes*. Oxford, Butterworth Heinemann.

McGee, P. and Castledine, G. (eds) (2003) *Advanced Nursing Practice*, 2nd edn. Oxford, Blackwell Publishing.

National Primary and Care Trust Development Programme (NATPACT) (2005) *Welcome to Action Learning*. www.natpact.nhs.uk (accessed 30/5/2007).

NHS Leadership Centre (2004) *Leadership and Race Equality: mentorship guidelines*. London, NHS Modernisation Agency.

Nursing and Midwifery Council (2006) *Standards to Support Learning and Assessment in Practice: NMC standards for mentors, practice teachers and teachers*. London, NMC.

Rolfe, G., Freshwater, D. and Jasper, M. (2001) *Critical Reflection for Nursing and the Helping Professions: a user's guide*. Basingstoke, Palgrave.

Thomas, J. and Etheridge, G. (2004) Using action learning to support and develop the role of matrons. *Nursing Times* 100, 34, 36–38.

Weinstein, K. (1999) *Action Learning: a practical guide*, 2nd edn. Aldershot, Gower.

10 Developing and sustaining professional partnerships

Julie Bliss

Introduction

The need for effective partnerships in health and social care delivery has been evident for a number of years. The central tenant of Partnership in Action (DH, 1998) was joint working and the need to work in partnership at three levels: strategic planning, service commissioning and service provision. Effective partnership working faces a multiplicity of challenges at organisational, professional and individual levels. However, focusing on the needs of the individual and their family does provide a common goal for all involved in care delivery and can facilitate partnership working (Cowley et al., 2002). The importance of joint working and partnership has not diminished with the move to practice-based commissioning; partnership is still key to health and social care policy (DH, 2006). The changing patterns of care delivery mean that individuals with multiple needs are increasingly being cared for within primary care; for these individuals disease-specific services may not address their needs (Lynch et al., 2005). Advanced community practitioners working as case managers will need to work in partnership with a variety of professionals across health, statutory and non-statutory organisations. In order to achieve this, it is important to understand the principles underpinning partnership working and consider the challenges and facilitators faced by professionals seeking to develop partnerships. This chapter explores these factors and considers how partnerships can be developed, maintained and evaluated.

REFLECTION: Critically consider your own experience of being involved with care delivery and identify the number of people involved in delivering a complex package of care (see also *Case study 10.1*).

Case study 10.1 Partnership working

Consider an 83-year-old patient who is severely disabled by arthritis. For the last three years she has had the same two unqualified formal carers provided by the local social services department, seven days each week, helping her with her hygiene needs. She lives alone and until recently her daughter, who lives 60 miles away, visited once a fortnight. She has recently been diagnosed with cancer of the liver and her condition is deteriorating rapidly. Her daughter is currently staying with her in the one-bedroomed flat. To ensure an effective care package is in place, a number of individuals will be involved, for example, the daughter, the district nurse, Macmillan nurse, GP, oncologist, social services and a Marie Curie nurse. Partnership working, between individuals, health and social care and a non-statutory organisation, is imperative.

Source: Bliss and While, 2003

Importance of partnership working

The value of working together is not a new concept, although it is only in the last 10 years or so that the phrase 'partnership working' has been used. The British Medical Association (BMA, 1965) introduced GP attachment, the Seebohm (1968) Report proposed closer collaboration between health and social care and the NHS and Community Care Act 1990 was based on collaboration as the cornerstone of providing holistic care with a minimal overlap of services. More recently the Health Committee (1998) found that collaboration will continue to present challenges while health and social care are not integrated. The Health Act 1999 moved towards integration by identifying pooled budgets, lead commissioning and integrated provision. The move to provide integrated care which meets the needs of individual service users is further addressed within the National Service Framework for Older People (DH, 2001) which introduced the single assessment process (SAP).

Interprofessional working is not only focused on health and social care but also plays a key role across the primary–secondary care interface. This is evidenced by the ongoing discussion regarding discharge planning. The Department of Health (2003) published a handbook for discharge which emphasised the importance of multi-professional and multiagency team working across the discharge process. Hospital discharge continues to be explored within the literature. Huby et al. (2007) undertook an ethnographic study in Scotland which identified varied practice. It was evident that where the team was actively engaged in interprofessional working it did have a positive impact on care delivery and discharge. The need for effective interprofessional and interagency working is not restricted to working with older people. *Working Together for Better Diabetes Care* (Roberts, 2007) provided illustrations of best practice, for example diabetes specialists working with primary care teams to set up diabetes clinics within GP surgeries. Roberts (2007) identified that partnership working, between clinicians and patients and across the primary–secondary care interface, is essential for people with diabetes.

The National Service Framework for Children, Young People and Maternity Services (DH, 2004) also promotes a change in service delivery, moving away from services focused on illnesses or problems but being child-centred, considering the child and the family. This acknowledges the challenges of caring for service users with complex needs, health, social care or education and reflects the challenges identified by Lynch et al. (2005) when caring for older people using disease-focused services. In order for services to be child-centred, there is an ongoing need for interprofessional working. The development of children's trusts may reduce some of the interagency challenges but effective partnerships are unlikely to be established without consideration of the multiple facets of collaboration and interprofessional working. Interprofessional and interagency working continues to be placed at the centre of healthcare provision. With *Creating a Patient-led NHS* (DH, 2005) calling for joined-up services to provide integrated care for patients with services spanning professional boundaries.

Despite the key role of interprofessional, interagency and partnership working in healthcare policy, there continues to be a lack of clarity regarding meaning and operationalisation. A documentary analysis by Mathew et al. (2003) found no evidence of consistent terminology regarding partnership working in palliative care policy documents, despite the increasing emphasis on partnership. This lack of consistent terminology and in consequence shared meaning in relation to interprofessional working has implications for effective palliative care delivery by professionals working across a variety of organisations, which include the NHS, local authority and the non-statutory sectors. Furthermore, the Continuing Care Report (House of Commons Health Committee, 2004–2005) noted disputes between health and social care provision, indicating that service provision remains fragmented despite the existence of policies to minimise this, for example, the single assessment process (DH, 2001) which sets out to reduce the plethora of assessments which take place for service users with complex needs. Taking these varied factors into consideration, it is important to understand what is meant by interprofessional working and the facilitators and challenges which impact on interprofessional working in order to be able to develop and sustain partnership working.

The variety of language used within policy documents and literature is one example of the challenges faced by professionals endeavouring to develop partnerships for care delivery. Interprofessional and multi-professional are often used interchangably. However, Davis (1988) proposed that multi-professional work acknowledges that others have a contribution to make; in contrast, Davis (1988) also suggested that interprofessional means that professionals are willing to work together to plan, deliver and evaluate care. While this may appear to be a debate focusing on semantics, it is an important philosophical difference that professionals need to embrace if partnership working is to be effective and sustainable. MacIntosh and McCormack (2001) clarify this difference further by identifying the different processes used to reach a common goal (see Figure 10.1).

Multi

Partners from different domains work independently to achieve a common purpose

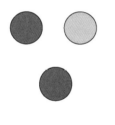

Multidisciplinary

Multi-sectoral   Multi-professional

Inter

Partners from different domains work interdependently to achieve a common purpose

Interdisciplinary   Intersectoral

Interprofessional

Figure 10.1 Different processes, common goal

Source: MacIntosh and McCormack, 2001: 549

The underpinning principle of interprofessional working is that of collaboration, a complex phenomenon open to various interpretations since it is variable. To develop effective partnership working a common understanding of collaboration is required. Henneman et al. (1995) undertook a concept analysis of collaboration that facilitated the defining attributes of collaboration (see Table 10.1).

Table 10.1 Defining attributes of collaboration

Joint venture	Cooperative endeavour
Willing participation	Shared planning and decision making
Team approach	Contribution of expertise
Shared responsibility	Non-hierarchical relationships
Power is shared: based on expertise knowledge and expertise versus role or title	

Source: Henneman et al., 1995: 105

For advanced practitioners working within primary care, these attributes are not immediately apparent and require practitioners to be proactive in order to achieve collaboration between professionals and the variety of organisations that provide care within primary care, for example social services, education, housing and the non-statutory sector such as Marie Curie. Multiple factors impact on an individual's ability to work as a team member and share decision making. It could be argued that within healthcare it is not possible to have non-hierarchical relationships and shared decision making. However, while some decisions are profession specific (Ovretveit, 1995), for example sectioning a mental health patient or registering a child at risk, everyone involved is able to contribute valuable information regarding the situation which should inform the decision. For example, on a stroke unit in Scotland a weekly meeting was held to discuss all inpatients (Huby et al., 2007) and provide an opportunity for members of the team to contribute their knowledge of the patient to the discussion. This information was then used by the consultant when deciding on the input from the team for future care delivery.

Collaboration can improve care for the patient and their family, for example patients with depression (Fickel et al., 2007). The positive impact interprofessional care delivery can have for the patient is a key driver that should promote willing participation by different professionals and organisations. However, before this and other defining attributes can be achieved it is important to consider factors that can facilitate and challenge collaboration and interprofessional working. A study to identify an effective model of shared care for service users with palliative care needs identified several factors which appeared to have contributed to a 'good' model of working together (Cowley et al., 2002). Four cases were investigated, which comprised a variety of community trusts, local authorities and specialist palliative care services. The case that did provide evidence of effective interprofessional working in part appeared to be a result of factors out of the control of the organisations. For example, the longevity of staff working together, a factor that cannot be imposed in practice but could be fostered by increased job satisfaction.

The suggestion that effective interprofessional working is fostered as a result of attitude, skill and culture rather than structural changes is supported by Kharicha et al. (2004). It is of interest to note that interprofessional working has been identified as one way of increasing job satisfaction since patients receive best quality care to meet their individual needs. Cowley et al. (2002) also identified that geography of the teams was important, for example, the health centre and social services office were on the same housing estate. Close geographical proximity is not always possible, furthermore community nurses and other nurse practitioners may work in multiple teams, which form in relation to the patient; this provides an additional degree of complexity to developing working relationships with other professionals. Taking into consideration that it is not always possible to reconfigure services to provide the perfect setting for interprofessional working and partnerships, it is crucial that advanced practitioners understand the principles of interprofessional working and the challenges that need to be considered if partnerships are to be developed and maintained.

> **REFLECTION:** Partnership working is central to delivering complex care packages and working across the primary–secondary care interface. Critically consider the defining attributes of collaboration in relation to your own practice and the organisation within which you work.

Influences of effective partnership working

There is a considerable amount of literature exploring team work, collaboration and interprofessional working. A recent review of the literature undertaken as part of a FrAmework for Multi-agency Environments (FAME), a national project led by local authorities (Gannon-Leary et al., 2006), identified four main themes: vision and engagement, governance, resources and capacity, people and practice. It is of interest to note the degree of overlap between each of these themes, which illustrates the fact that interprofessional working, and thus partnership working, is influenced by individuals, organisations and policy. In order to explore these areas it is helpful to consider examples from practice. While Cowley et al. (2002) identified a 'good' model of shared care for service users with palliative care needs, palliative care provides an interesting example of the challenges faced when working in partnership to deliver quality care. Palliative care requires management of both physical and psychosocial symptoms in order to meet complex care needs, furthermore to achieve this it may also be necessary to work across organisational boundaries (Bliss et al., 2000). Therefore, palliative care provides a vehicle to explore interprofessional working in relation to the organisations and the professionals involved in care delivery.

Bliss (2007) explored the different ways in which district nurses and social workers work, both interprofessionally and with service users when providing packages of palliative and continuing care. In each case, minimal evidence of direct interactions between the district nurse and social worker was found, despite the evidence that communication is important if interprofessional working is to be effective (While and Barriball, 1999). The district nurses and social workers both placed the service user at the centre of care provision suggesting a common goal. However, this was operationalised in different ways.

The district nurses undertook the initial assessment for all of the referrals and revisited the service user as the care package was set up, thereby continuing to play an active role over a number of visits and developing the assessment. In contrast, social workers completed the assessment of those identified by clerical staff as having complex needs (Bliss, 2007), social workers conducted the assessment during one visit and then organised the care package. This disparity in the management of initial assessments is potentially a source of conflict within the single assessment process (DH, 2001) and illustrates one aspect for consideration with regards to partnership working. It is important to understand that the underpinning philosophy and processes by which different professional groups work may differ. Understanding these differences can contribute to the development of common understandings and goals, which have been found to be key to interprofessional working (Cowley et al., 2002; Sheehan et al., 2007)

The district nurses were concerned with maintaining optimum well-being for the service users; in contrast, the social workers took a pragmatic approach focusing on activities of daily living and maintaining service users in their own homes (Bliss, 2007). Worth (2001) identified that social workers experienced a reduction of case work and therapeutic interventions with service users following the move to care management. This may inhibit service users benefiting from the skills and expertise of social workers, it is important to have a working knowledge of the skills and expertise of different professional groups if there is to be an effective contribution of expertise, a defining attribute of collaboration (Henneman et al., 1995).

While exploring district nurses' and social workers' ways of working it was identified that the district nurses were more likely to advocate a change in the place of care than the social workers. Funding issues may have impacted on the place of care delivery; district nurses are able to access care, such as a hospice bed, free at the point of delivery. In contrast, social workers manage the cost implications of care packages directly. The different organisational constraints in relation to palliative care delivery across organisations have been explored in more detail by Bliss et al. (2000). Funding and resources continue to be a key factor in partnership working. Christensen and Roberts (2005) found that means testing was a source of tension for district nurses involved in the single assessment process.

While this exploration of the ways in which district nurses and social workers work within their organisations contributes to an understanding of some of the potential different ways of working it would be an error to assume that if professionals work within the same organisation these challenges no longer exist. Henneman et al. (1995) identified the importance of the professionals' understanding of their own role in order to work collaboratively. If professionals are not able to articulate their role it is difficult for other professional groups to make appropriate referrals and use the expertise available. Bliss (1998) explored district nurses and social worker understanding of one another's role. It was of interest to note that within the six district nurses there was dissonance regarding role, for example, in relation to taking blood. The challenge of role understanding has not diminished, neither is it restricted to health. An exploration of professional relationships between health and social care when working with frail older people found that the social workers felt that care management was nebulous, potentially removing 'real' social work, to the point that one social worker felt unable to articulate their role (Hudson, 2002). While professionals may have an understanding of part of the role of other professional groups, for example, social workers referring to the district nursing service for medication management, unless roles and expertise are clearly articulated service users may not receive the full benefit of utilising skill mix in order to provide quality care packages.

Bliss (1998) also identified examples of the challenge of language, for example, the social worker was unsure what a suprapubic catheter was and felt that the district nurse should care for it, in contrast the district nurse felt that the formal carer could manage it with a weekly visit from the district nursing team. One method of overcoming the difficulty of language and communication is to meet and discuss individuals and their care needs. The communication network between professionals and service users was identified as an important facilitator of interprofessional working in a 'good' model of palliative care (Cowley et al., 2002). Despite the consensus that communication networks are important, achieving good practice, effective communication remains a challenge. For example, from a sample of eight service users receiving district nurse and social work input only three case conferences took place during the data collection period (Bliss, 2007). For practitioners working in multiple teams, who may be geographically apart and within different organisations, regular communication is a challenge that must not be ignored. With regards to individuals and their care package this can be achieved by a key worker to facilitate continuity of care (Cowley et al., 2002).

> **REFLECTION:** Given the variety of factors that impact on partnership working, critically examine your own working practice and organisation. Consider if any changes in working could further enhance partnership working.

Developing new partnerships

Consideration of the multiplicity of factors that impact on interprofessional working and the consequences of these factors on patient care is not sufficient to ensure effective partnership working. This chapter has examined some of influences on partnership working at an individual, professional and organisational level. It could be argued that as a result of the many faceted challenges, partnership working is a Utopian dream. However, as previously discussed, the benefits for service users mean that partnership working is a goal worthy of achievement. Indeed, it is impossible to work in isolation when providing care for service users with complex needs, the service users most likely to be in receipt of care from the variety of advanced nurse practitioners involved in care delivery. The NHS Modernisation Agency and Skills for Health (2005) identified the need for coordinated care for service users with complex care needs, a recurrent theme that remains central to quality care delivery. The competency framework for case management clearly identifies the importance of interagency and partnership working within the key domains. This reinforces the need for advanced practitioners to be proactive to establish a good understanding of the different roles and expertise of professionals involved in care delivery and the varied organisations within which they work. For example, a patient with complex needs may receive input from the community matron, the GP, the hospital consultant, the pharmacist and social services. Within the range of professionals there are two healthcare organisations (primary care trust, acute trust), two independent businesses (GP and pharmacist) and local authority provision. The need to work effectively with this range of professionals is evident in the literature previously discussed with regards to making use of expert knowledge to deliver quality care. One example of this is prescribing: it is impossible to prescribe without considering the interface between prescribers, understanding the functions and role of team members and sharing information with the team (NMC, 2005).

Perhaps the most important consideration for advanced practitioners in relation to partnership working is the importance of leadership within the role. It is not sufficient to focus on the delivery of care if advanced practitioners are to be proactive in developing partnership working. The NHS Institute for Innovation and Improvement (2003) sets out the qualities required in order to develop services and deliver care. Parallels can be drawn between the personal qualities identified and the antecedents for collaboration (Henneman et al., 1995), for example, self-belief and awareness and confidence in role and expertise. The drive for improvement, a personal quality identified by the leadership qualities framework is a central tenant of interprofessional working, effective partnership, interagency working and community involvement. The proactive advanced practitioner will need to understand the issues within their own organisation as well as across health and social care. The importance of collaboration is apparent within the leadership qualities framework which identifies collaboration as a key quality with regards to delivering the service (NHS Institute for Innovation and Improvement, 2003).

Advanced practitioners need to be forging long-term partnerships, thereby working at the highest level of leadership with regards to collaboration. While an understanding of the challenges of interprofessional working is helpful when developing partnership working, Hardy et al. (2003) have developed an assessment tool that can be used to facilitate an appraisal of effectiveness of partnership working in practice. The tool was developed by the Strategic Partnership Taskforce of the Office of the Deputy Prime Minister, which was established to identify innovative ways in which local government could develop public services by utilising effective partnership working. The tool is based on six principles of partnership working identified by research and as such provides guiding principles for advanced nurse practitioners involved in developing partnerships (see Table 10.2). These principles are supported by the focus on individual service user need as a common goal which engenders partnership working at a case level and can be further developed across professional groups and different organisations.

> **REFLECTION:** Having considered ways of enhancing partnership working consider your own leadership style and how you can work within the organisation to take this forward.

Table 10.2 The six partnership principles

Principle 1: Recognise and accept the need for partnership
Principle 2: Develop clarity and realism of purpose
Principle 3: Ensure commitment and ownership
Principle 4: Develop and maintain trust
Principle 5: Create clear and robust partnership arrangements
Principle 6: Monitor, measure and learn

Source: Hardy et al., 2003: 14

Sustaining and evaluating partnership working

The most immediate evaluation of partnership working is the output of the partnership with regards to the quality of care provision for individual service users and their families. However, the multiple demands faced by individuals and organisations involved in care delivery are many and varied, for example, reduction of bed days and means-tested service delivery. These challenges may mean that the individual service user's need may not be the central focus of interprofessional working for all involved. It is at this point that advanced nurse practitioners and their role as care coordinators play a key role in maintaining the focus of partnership working on the package of care for the service user. The partnership assessment tool (Hardy et al., 2003) provides a vehicle to identify the strengths and challenges of a specific partnership. The assessment is completed individually by all involved in the partnership, the scores are then collated and the aggregate score for each principle can be identified. This facilitates the identification of areas which may need further work, for example developing and maintaining trust, an antecedent to collaborative working (Henneman et al., 1995). Evaluating the effectiveness of partnership working does not need to be complex; indeed, Henneman et al. (1995) identified that if collaboration is in place there will be increased dialogue between the team, interprofessional standards and perhaps more importantly the use of 'we' statements as opposed to 'I' statements.

Summary

Rushmer and Pallis (2002) were clear that working together is not about blurring boundaries but about each professional making a unique contribution. Policy, empirical studies and anecdotal evidence all support the view that partnership working is key to the delivery of quality care. Advanced practitioners are ideally placed to develop and sustain partnerships both at an individual and organisational level. It is imperative that consideration is given to the interprofessional issues, such as understanding of role, language and communication, as well as the organisational considerations such as funding, hierarchies and philosophical differences. However, advanced practitioners must remember that the leadership qualities framework (NHS Institute for Innovation and Improvement, 2003) identifies the personal qualities required for effective partnership working and furthermore that interpersonal skills are key to effective partnerships. This chapter has explored the challenges of partnership working in primary care, these challenges may be compounded by the move to primary care trusts, commissioning, rather than providing services. With the increase in providers, it is imperative that advanced nurse practitioners have a clear understanding of effective partnership working.

References

Bliss, J. (1998) District nurses' and social workers' understanding of each other's role. *British Journal of Community Nursing* 3, 330–336.

Bliss, J. (2007) District nursing and social work: palliative and continuing care delivery. *British Journal of Community Nursing* 12, 268–272.

Bliss, J., Cowley, S. and While, A. (2000) Interprofessional working in palliative care in the community: a review of the literature. *Journal of Interprofessional Care* 14, 281–290.

Bliss, J. and While, A. (2003) Decision-making in palliative and continuing care in the community: an analysis of the published literature with reference to the context of UK care provision. *International Journal of Nursing Studies* 40, 881–888.

British Medical Association (BMA) (1965) *Charter for the Family Doctor Service*. London, BMA.

Christensen, A. and Roberts, K. (2005) Integrating health and social care assessment and care management: findings from a pilot project evaluation. *Primary Health Care Research and Development* 6, 269–277.

Cowley, S., Bliss, J., Mathew, A. and McVey, G. (2002) Effective interagency and interprofessional working: facilitators and barriers. *International Journal of Palliative Nursing* 8, 30–39.

Davis, C. (1988) Philosophical foundations of interdisciplinarity in caring for the elderly, or the willingness to change your mind. *Physiotherapy Practice* 4, 23–25.

Department of Health (DH) (1998) *Partnership in action: new opportunities for joint working between health and social services*. London, DH.

Department of Health (DH) (2001) *National Service Framework for Older People*. London, DH.

Department of Health (DH) (2003) *Discharge from hospital: pathway, process and practice*. London, DH.

Department of Health (DH) (2004) *National Service Framework for Children, Young People and Maternity Services.* London, DH.

Department of Health (DH) (2005) *Creating a Patient-led NHS.* London, DH.

Department of Health (DH) (2006) *Our Health, Our Care, Our Say: a new direction for community services Cm 6737.* London, HMSO.

Fickel, J., Parker, L., Yano E. and Kirchner, J. (2007) Primary care – mental health collaboration: an example of assessing usual practice and potential barriers. *Journal of Interprofessional Care* 21, 207–216.

Gannon-Leary, P., Baines, S. and Wilson, R. (2006) Collaboration and partnership: a review and reflections on a national project to join up local services in England. *Journal of Interprofessional Care* 20, 665–674.

Hardy, B., Hudson, B. and Waddington, E. (2003) *Assessing Strategic Partnership: the partnership assessment tool.* London, Office of the Deputy Prime Minister.

Health Act (1999) *Chapter 8.* London, The Stationery Office.

Health Committee (1998) *The Relationship between Health and Social Services.* London, The Stationery Office.

Henneman, E., Lee, J. and Cohen, J. (1995) Collaboration: a concept analysis. *Journal of Advanced Nursing* 21, 103–109.

House of Commons Health Committee (2004–2005) *Sixth Report NHS Continuing Care HC 399–1.* London, The Stationery Office.

Huby, G., Holt Brook, J., Thompson, A. and Tierney, A. (2007) Capturing the concealed: interprofessional practice and older peoples' participation in decision-making about discharge after acute hospitalisation. *Journal of interprofessional Care* 21, 55–67.

Hudson, B. (2002) Interprofessionality in health and social care: the Achilles' heel of partnership. *Journal of Interprofessional Care* 16, 7–17.

Kharicha, K., Levin, E., Iliffe, S. and Davey, B. (2004) Social work, general practice and evidence-based policy in collaborative care of older people: current problems and future possibilities. *Health & Social Care in the Community* 12, 134–141.

Lynch, M., Estes, C. and Henandez, M. (2005) Chronic care initiatives for the elderly: can they bridge the gerontology-medicine gap? *Journal of Applied Gerontology* 24, 108–124.

MacIntosh, J. and McCormack, D. (2001) Partnerships identified within primary health care literature. *International Journal of Nursing Studies* 38, 547–555.

Mathew, A., Cowley, S., Bliss, J. and Thistlewood, G. (2003) The development of palliative care in national government policy in England 1986–2000. *Palliative Medicine* 17, 270–282.

NHS and Community Care Act (1990) London, HMSO.

NHS Institute for Innovation and Improvement (2003) *The NHS Leadership Qualities Framework.* London, NHS Institute for Innovation and Improvement.

NHS Modernisation Agency and Skills for Health (2005) *Case Management Competency Framework.* London, NHS Modernisation Agency, Skills for Health.

Nursing and Midwifery Council (NMC) (2005) *Standards for the Proficiency for Nurse and Midwife Prescribers*. London, NMC.

Ovretveit, J. (1995) Team decision making. *Journal of Interprofessional Care* 9, 41–51.

Roberts, S. (2007) *Working Together for Better Diabetes Care*. London, DH.

Rushmer, R. and Pallis, G. (2002) Inter-professional working: the wisdom of integrated working and the disaster of blurred boundaries. *Public Money and Management*, 59–66.

Seebohm, F. (1968) *The Report of the Committee on Local Authority and Personal Social Services*. London, HMSO.

Sheehan, D., Robertson, L. and Ormond, T. (2007) Comparison of language and patterns of communication in interprofessional and multidisciplinary teams. *Journal of interprofessional Care* 21, 17–30.

While, A. and Barriball, L. (1999) Qualified and unqualified nurses' views of the multidisciplinary team: findings of a large interview study. *Journal of Interprofessional Care* 13, 77–90.

Worth, A. (2001) Assessment of needs of older people by district nurses and social workers: a changing culture? *Journal of interprofessional Care* 15, 257–266.

11 From involvement to partnerships and beyond

Ian Price

What is false in the science of facts may be true in the science of values.
Santayana (1900)

Power is the ability to define phenomena and have them react accordingly.
Huey P. Newton, co-founder of the Black Panther Party

Introduction

The development of patient and public involvement in the National Health Service is arguably the most significant aspect of recent government health policy. Over the past 30 years or more there have been many attempts to reorganise the structure and management of the NHS with varying degrees of success. Although the drive towards what has come to be termed a patient-led NHS has also been accompanied by such a restructuring, the aim of policy to ensure that the public is at the heart of all NHS activity at all levels (DH, 2001) has the potential to outlast the effects of organisational reconfigurations. These policy initiatives both reflect and reinforce the development of wider societal consumerist attitudes and the consequent differing expectations of the nature of the relationship between service providers and the public.

The importance of patient and public involvement in primary care is highlighted by the World Health Organisation (1978) which sees community involvement in the development, implementation and evaluation of services as crucial. Government policy in the UK has reflected this to an increasing extent since the Community Care Act 1990, which required the commissioning of services that reflected the views and needs of the local population and involved users in evaluating the success of these services.

The nature and extent of policy initiatives relating to this aspect of public sector provision (and in many ways beyond) have been vast. The drive towards a patient-led NHS (DH, 2005) encompasses a range of both strategic and operational activities at many different levels with the NHS. For practitioners the main consequence of these developments is the need to work in a way that encompasses the concept of user involvement. (Note that the term 'user involvement' is often extended to 'user and carer involvement'. This discussion, however, is confined to issues relating to the former term. It is recognised that although the two activities are often conflated, there are distinct issues that need to be considered when discussing carer involvement that are beyond the scope of this chapter.)

The phrase user involvement initially became popular in the field of mental health as result of the growth of the user movement and, despite a degree of controversy surrounding the term, it has also gained currency in other areas of health and social care. The growth of user involvement has been associated with the increase in consumerism in society generally but the characteristics and scope of user involvement currently being advocated within policy go beyond a narrow definition of consumerism to encompass a much wider definition that embraces real democratic empowerment and engagement of communities. The nuances of the definition will be discussed in more detail later in the chapter but, broadly speaking, the term is used to encompass a range of activities that require actual or potential end users of health and social care services to have active participation in all aspects of their care.

Traditional interpretations of professional behaviour and of that expected of the public when accessing professional help stress very clear predetermined and hierarchical functions for both parties. Effective and meaningful user involvement requires more flexible and responsive behaviours from the professional within the context of a more egalitarian relationship and interaction. While this is obviously concerned with doing things differently (or perhaps more accurately, doing different things), effective user involvement also requires from practitioners a different set of attitudes and values. The need for the development of such attitudes and values will be discussed more fully later in the chapter but it is worth noting at this point that effective user involvement requires a professional commitment both to such participation and to changes in behaviour underpinned by an understanding of the reasons why such practice is necessary.

Concept of user involvement

The concept of user involvement is problematic. As is often the case, the initial difficulty concerns terminology. A cursory examination of the literature reveals a number of terms that are closely related and often not clearly defined or differentiated from one another. For example, Cahill (1998) suggests that from a nursing perspective 'patient participation' is a vague and poorly described term and also describes the same term as 'over-used and ambiguous' (Cahill, 1996). To some extent, this reflects the use of different language in different areas of health or social care but whatever the reason for the confusion it is important to be able to define clearly what is being discussed.

The first challenge relates to describing *who* is being involved. The literature commonly employs terms such as clients, users, the public and patients (notwithstanding the difficulties of using the last term with its traditional associations of passivity in connection with active involvement). For the purposes of this discussion, the term user involvement will be used, other than when referring to terms quoted in specific sources. In adopting this term, it is recognised that this is not without its own attendant difficulties and that many practitioners will be uncomfortable with its use.

Literature relating to user involvement also commonly refers to concepts such as patient participation, collaboration, patient involvement, patient partnership, as well as shared decision making and person-centred planning (Millard et al., 2006). Government policy also refers to a patient-led NHS and to patient and public involvement (DH, 2001, 2005). In order to begin to address some of the potential confusion surrounding these terms, a clear distinction between 'patient' and 'public' needs to be made.

Poulton (1999) describes how user involvement is used to describe a wide variety of interactions and relationships between healthcare providers and those who use such services. Although acknowledging that these encompass a range of activities, she divides such involvement into two broad types: activities that develop the ability of services to meet the needs of individuals; and strategic means of increasing the influence of users in the design, management and review of services. This distinction is echoed by Florin and Dixon (2004) who describe *public* involvement [sic] as participation, either at a local or national level, in strategic determination of policy or service. They distinguish this from *patient* participation which they describe as decisions made by individual patients about their own care in conjunction with health professionals. It is this distinction that government policy also explicitly makes clear (DH, 2004). The difference between involvement at the individual or operational level and that undertaken at the strategic level is important as it requires practitioners not only to recognise that such a distinction exists but also be able to function effectively at both these levels.

If there is, therefore, a degree of certainty about the difference between patient and public (or potential patients') involvement, can we be equally certain that we understand what is meant by terms such as involvement, collaboration, participation and partnership? Indeed, do we need to concern ourselves with discussing definitions of such terms or do they all essentially mean the same?

A detailed examination of the finer nuances of definition of each of these terms is beyond the scope of this discussion; however, a basic understanding of some distinctions between the words as used in this context is essential to ensure that practitioners are able to locate their practice appropriately within the range of possible actions implied by each term.

It is also probable that, as we examine the distinctions between such terms in increasing depth, a diversity of opinions will be revealed and achieving a consensus will become increasingly contentious and problematic. As we have seen, terms have been poorly defined and over-used in the past (Cahill, 1996, 1998) and although there has been some progress more recently in understanding what these terms represent, further clarification is still necessary.

One means by which greater clarity might be achieved is to consider the terms as a hierarchy of actions or as points along a continuum. Millard et al. (2006), for example, argue that terms are not synonymous and therefore are not interchangeable and describe patient involvement/collaboration, patient participation and patient partnership, in ascending order, as distinct hierarchical activities. Poulton (1999) also describes a hierarchy beginning with information at the base and culminating in empowerment at the top which encompasses (among other activities) health education, consultation and participation. Moving up the hierarchy requires a change in the nature and an increase in the degree of involvement required of the recipient.

This has echoes in the participation continuum described by Hickey and Kipping (1998). They propose four distinct points on the continuum: information/explanation, consultation, partnership and user control. Although specifically addressing mental health services, they also usefully add a factor to their continuum which helps highlight the possible tensions between the driving forces behind user involvement. They categorise information/explanation and consultation as reflective of a consumerist approach to user involvement. This increases choice through more responsive reactions to expressed preferences but is merely concerned about what is good or bad about services as they stand and does not in any way challenge the underlying ideology of service provision. Partnership and user control, by way of contrast, are seen by Hickey and Kipping (1998) as characterising a democratisation approach to user involvement. This has wider implications than a consumerist approach in that it sees individuals not only as users of services but also as 'citizens' who have a right to be involved in decisions not only about their individual care but also about service configuration (Hickey and Kipping, 1998).

The points on the continuum described by Hickey and Kipping (1998) can be seen as broadly comparable to but not directly analogous to those concepts described by Cahill (1996, 1998), Poulton (1999) and Millard et al. (2006). Information/explanation and consultation are characterised by the one-way flow of information (from professional to user) identified by Poulton (1999) and the possibility that the voice of the user can be ignored as highlighted by Cahill (1996, 1998) and Poulton (1999). Such an approach also does not require any narrowing of the knowledge gap between professional and public. In terms of democratisation, partnership as described by Hickey and Kipping (1998) is closer to the participation described by Cahill (1996) and Poulton (1999) in that it involves users in direct decision making at both an individual and collective level.

This distinction between consumerist and democratisation approaches to user involvement helps make clearer the move from the consumerist approach that initially drove the move towards user involvement during the 1980s to the democratisation that now appears to underpin the political imperative for a patient-led NHS. The distinction also highlights the need for a fundamentally different way of understanding and acting within the context of the relationship between professionals and the public.

Hickey and Kipping (1998) perhaps go further than either Cahill or Poulton in identifying the potential extent of user involvement in that they explicitly refer to user *control* (emphasis added), characterised by a redistribution of power so that users make decisions, including whether to involve others (professionals included). This is probably more reflective of the concepts underpinning the patient-led NHS than participation as described by Cahill (1996) and this difference is in all likelihood reflective of the differing rates of progress in the degree of user involvement within different care contexts over the past 10 years. Poulton (1999), however, comes closer to the idea of user control in terms of describing the highest level of involvement although this stops short of user control as empowerment is described as power sharing *with* professionals.

It appears, therefore, that many terms are used to describe the concept of user involvement and although there probably remains some confusion in some quarters there is also a degree of consensus emerging from the literature.

Relationship between the professional and user

Whatever term is used to describe user involvement, one aspect of the activity emerges clearly from the literature as being crucial to its success. This is the relationship between the professional and the user, variously described as a distinctive, consistent and fundamental feature of user involvement (Cahill, 1996; Millard et al., 2006) and a prerequisite for effective participation (Sahlsten et al., 2005). The relationship is the means by which effective communication and the imparting of information takes place with the consequent shift in power to the user (Sahlsten et al., 2005; Millard et al., 2006). Cahill (1996) emphasises that the degree of patient participation is dependent on the quality and depth of the relationship. It appears, therefore, that this interaction is at the heart and crucial to the success of user involvement and that the professional's actions within this are critical.

Millard et al. (2006) have proposed an involving/non-involving continuum for considering how helpful professional actions are within this relationship in fostering effective involvement. This provides a useful framework for practitioners to reflect on their actions and make judgements about the effectiveness of their actions. The continuum begins with behaviours that are described as *non-involving*, characterised by the user not being invited to participate in decision making at all even after the professional becomes aware of the user's opinions. This behaviour can be either overt or covert. *Forced involving* describes situations where the professional calls on the user to play a part in decision making only after being challenged by the user to do so. *Partially involving* behaviours occur when the user is asked to participate in decision making about some aspects of care and the continuum is completed by *completely involving* behaviours when the user is invited to participate in decision making about all aspects of their care (Millard et al., 2006).

Professional behaviour is obviously a critical factor in determining where along this continuum participation can be said to occur and Millard et al. (2006) further identify four sub-properties of this behaviour. These are open/closed interactive approach, patient/task focus, inclusive/exclusive style and full/no reciprocity. They also suggest that behaviours which can be described as completely involving focus not only on the professional dimension of the relationship (i.e. that related to the patient's illness and care) but also extend into the social dimension, which entail personal communication beyond that appropriate to everyday conversation (Millard et al., 2006).

Sahlsten et al. (2005) take this idea further by proposing that therapeutic behaviour requires a genuine interest in the patient which is characterised by empathetic understanding, sincerity and self-knowledge. Wilson (1999) supports this by reporting that people with long-term conditions want relationships based on mutual trust and respect. This has also been highlighted by a report from the Department of Health (2003) which emphasises the importance of patients' emotional experience and the role that professionals can play in addressing this. The notion that an effective relationship can in itself be therapeutic is not new to nursing as this was a central tenet of primary nursing as originally developed in the 1980s. However, the attention to the nurses' own attitudes and the effects that these have on actions has more recent echoes in the concept of values-based practice originally developed in child and adolescent services in mental health. The central role of the consideration of values in determining the effectiveness of this relationship will be addressed later in the chapter.

Attitudes and behaviour

If, from a theoretical perspective, professional attitudes and behaviour are crucial to the success of user involvement, ironically, arguably the single most critical factor mitigating against the development of user involvement in health and social care is the professional frame of mind towards patients. Traditionally, patients have been excluded both collectively and individually at all levels from decisions involving the design and delivery of services (Henderson, 2003). The paternalistic stance adopted by professionals traditionally saw patients as objects or bodies requiring surveillance or monitoring, as passive recipients of care and treatment (Cahill, 1998). Any move towards greater user involvement in aspects of planning and delivery must therefore address this attitude.

Attitudes to greater involvement have been described as mixed (Cahill, 1998). Professionals frequently feel threatened by an increase in the power wielded by patients and are often reluctant to relinquish power or control which is seen as an inevitable corollary of greater power in the hands of patients. One common reason for this professional protectionism (Poulton, 1999) is that patients are thought to be unable to understand information usually seen as the preserve of professionals (Cahill, 1998). The fear of increasing user expectations and consequently creating greater pressure on already stretched services have also been identified as factors inhibiting professional commitment to user involvement (Poulton, 1999). Negative attitudes to greater involvement are also linked to a lack of awareness or understanding of the driving forces behind such a move. Conversely, enthusiasm for and a commitment to greater patient involvement are related to positive individual values held by the professional (Cahill, 1998).

Poulton (1999) has characterised the different perceptions of what characterises good care and effective services between professionals and users in primary care as a 'cultural divide' and that narrowing this requires active facilitation. However, Clough (2003) highlights that both parties experience genuine anxieties as a result of increased user involvement and that these must be acknowledged and addressed. Some of the anxieties felt by professionals may well emanate from an uncertainty (and consequent anxiety about) of what is required of them in the context of increased user involvement. Indeed, both parties in the undertaking might be unclear about what is expected of them and how this might be achieved. A discussion of what preparation the public requires in order to be able to participate effectively in such a context is beyond the scope of this chapter but there are some crucial changes to professional roles that must be understood if professionals are to avoid the current mistake of assuming that they are involving users when they are not (Clough, 2003)!

Clough (2003) argues that professionals (he is writing about medical staff but the point applies equally to all groups) must understand that greater user involvement requires a shift from acting as paternalistic 'expert advisors'. Defining patient needs independently of eliciting what these might be from the patient themselves, giving advice, solving problems, only passing on information considered to be appropriate by the professional and consequently increasing dependency are not practices that will correspond to users' expectations. What is required is partnership characterised by eliciting the needs from users, discussing options and jointly exploring solutions. This involves sharing all relevant information and in theory results in users that are empowered and enabled to participate fully in their care. This process, together with the development of an effective working relationship, could be facilitated by the use of an approach described as values-based practice.

Values-based practice

Originally developed by Fulford and Williams (2003) in the field of child and adolescent mental health services, this approach requires that values should explicitly be considered when determining professional actions and that appropriate values are developed to enable specific policy imperatives to be achieved. Values are deeply held views and guiding principles that can function at both an organisational and individual level (Pendleton and King, 2002). Sackett et al. (2000) have defined patients' values as the individual's unique preferences, concerns and expectations that must explicitly be considered to ensure that decisions made concerning care and treatment serve the interests of the user. Values can also be described as a filter through which the evidence used to underpin decisions concerning care and treatment is viewed (Lockwood, 2004) and it is probable that users and practitioners will have differing opinions as to the extent to which this evidence applies.

Values-based practice proceeds from the presumption of a diversity of equally legitimate values and that in many circumstances there may be no 'right' answer for all involved. This shifts the emphasis away from the 'right' outcome to consideration of what constitutes 'good process' in terms of decision making (Fulford and Williams, 2003). There is also explicit acknowledgement that all decisions are based on values as well as facts or evidence. Values-based and evidence-based practice are complementary rather than antagonistic to each other and in order for appropriate decisions to be made both values and evidence need to be considered (Fulford and Williams, 2003).

The framework, further developed by Williams (2005), defines values-based practice as an attempt to reconcile best research evidence with practitioner expertise and patient values through the development of a 'therapeutic alliance' which ensures the best possible 'clinical outcomes' and 'quality of life' (Williams, 2005). However, we only tend to become aware of values when these are diverse or conflicting. In these circumstances the need to incorporate values into decision making becomes potentially problematic.

Values-based practice requires that the 'first-call' for information is the point of view of the patient (Williams, 2005). This must also take into consideration the patient's wider familial context. Decisions are therefore made in a manner that allows for a balance of reasonably different values rather than by reference to a 'rule' that prescribes a 'right' outcome (Fulford and Williams, 2003) and this in turn requires greater attention to the process by which decisions are made, allowing appropriate decisions when values are not shared or where consensus is not immediately apparent.

Values-based practice, if not requiring a wholly new set of skills and knowledge of practitioners, does at the very least require the use of existing skills towards a different purpose. The adoption of this approach as a means of achieving user involvement requires increased understanding of the origins and nature of values and efforts to obtain as much information as is possible concerning the values that may have an influence on a specific decision. Fulford and Williams (2003) suggest that as well as traditional methods of acquiring such information (e.g. research or philosophical enquiry) less traditional means might also be employed; these would include study of literary sources and the consideration of user narratives. This would have the effect of reducing 'values myopia' (Fulford and Williams, 2003), the inclination to presuppose that values are shared. Greater exploration and consequent increased awareness and knowledge of values, however, will not eradicate differences and communication skills are crucial in achieving acceptable solutions. Patient perspective skills, listening to and exploring values, are crucial in being able to increase awareness and knowledge and negotiation and conflict resolution are necessary in order to be able to determine what to do where there are conflicting values (Fulford and Williams, 2003).

It is through the use of these skills that a change in the locus of control within decision making is reached. Within values-based practice, the process of providing an answer to the question 'who decides' evolves from the assumptions contained within the framework, namely values are diverse and increasingly influential and that the values of users are the dominant, although crucially, not the only perspective that needs to be incorporated into any course of action. Therefore, it is the users and practitioners at the 'clinical coal face' who decide.

REFLECTION: Look at the participation continuum shown in Figure 11.1:

- Where would you place your own practice on this? Why? Where do you think you should be?
- How do you feel about greater user involvement?
- Within your own practice, what factors inhibit or promote the level of user involvement?
- What values do you hold about the nature of your relationship with

users? Do you share these values with your colleagues? To what extent are these explicitly reflected in your practice?

- What part do your own behaviours play in determining the position you have identified on this continuum? How helpful are your professional actions are in fostering effective involvement with reference to the involving/non-involving continuum and its sub-properties as described by Millard et al. (2006).
- What steps do you take to ascertain the preferences, concerns and expectations of users? What factors influence the extent to which you consider these when making decisions concerning care and treatment that serve the interests of the user? When you are aware that your values and those of the user differ, what steps do you take to reconcile these differences?
- What values do you need to develop and what skills and knowledge do you need to acquire to increase the level of user involvement in your practice?

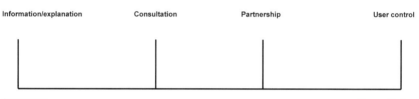

Figure 11.1 Participation continuum

Source: Hickey and Kipping, 1998

Summary

User involvement will, to a great extent, be achieved by the creation of mechanisms that allow patient and public contributions to local and national strategic and operational decision making from within the managerial structures of the NHS rather from without, as has been the case in the past (DH, 2001). However, user involvement also requires not just a set of actions on behalf of practitioners that allow such participation but nothing more than a reconceptualising, a rethinking, of the nature of their relationship with the public. This does not necessarily reflect a stance that is antagonistic to or incompatible with professional practice or professionals (although some of the more extreme manifestations of the user movement have stemmed from such a point of view) but it does require a different way of thinking about what it means to be a professional and professional action. Although the drive towards user involvement is not a direct challenge to professionalism per se, it is a challenge to certain models of professionalism and behaviours associated with these.

As the growth of patient and public involvement in the NHS is indicative of a shift in attitudes generally any attempt to remove or appreciably weaken these in the future will be difficult to achieve. If this is the case and such involvement becomes an entrenched part of the NHS, this would in part reflect achievement of the aim of shifting power and resources to the people for whom the service is provided in partnership with frontline staff (DH, 2001).

References

Cahill, J. (1996) Patient participation: a concept analysis. *Journal of Advanced Nursing* 24, 3, 561–571.

Cahill, J. (1998) Patient participation – a review of the literature. *Journal of Clinical Nursing* 7, 2, 119–128.

Clough, C. (2003) Involving patients and the public in the NHS. *Clinical Medicine* 3, 6, 551–554.

Department of Health (DH) (2001) *Involving Patients and the Public in Healthcare. A discussion document*. London, DH.

Department of Health (DH) (2003) *Results from a Programme of Consultation to Develop a Patient Experience Statement*. London, DH.

Department of Health (DH) (2004) *Patient and Public Involvement in Health: the evidence for policy implementation. A summary of the results of the Health in Partnership research programme*. London, DH.

Department of Health (DH) (2005) *Creating a Patient-led NHS: delivering the NHS improvement plan*. London, DH.

Florin, D. and Dixon, J. (2004) Public involvement in health care. *British Medical Journal* 328, 159–161.

Fulford, K. W. M. and Williams, R. (2003) Values-based child and adolescent mental health services? *Current Opinion in Psychiatry* 16, 369–376.

Henderson, S. (2003) Power imbalance between nurses and patients: a potential inhibitor of partnership in care. *Journal of Clinical Nursing* 12, 4, 501–508.

Hickey, G. and Kipping, C. (1998) Exploring the concept of user involvement in mental health through a participation continuum. *Journal of Clinical Nursing* 7, 1, 83–88.

Lockwood, S. (2004) Evidence of 'me' in evidence-based medicine? *British Medical Journal* 329, 1033–1035.

Millard, L., Hallett, C. and Luker, K. (2006) Nurse-patient interaction and decision-making in care: patient involvement in community nursing. *Journal of Advanced Nursing* 55, 2, 142–150.

Pendleton, D. and King, J. (2002) Values and leadership. *British Medical Journal* 325, 1352–1355.

Poulton, B. (1999) User involvement in identifying health needs and shaping services: is it being realised? *Journal of Advanced Nursing* 30, 6, 1289–1296.

Sackett, D. L., Straus, S. E. and Scott Richardson, W. (2000) *Evidence-based Medicine: how to practise and teach EBM*, 2nd edn. Edinburgh, Churchill Livingstone.

Sahlsten, M. J. M., Larsson, I. E., Lindencrona, C. S. C. and Plos, K. A. E. (2005) Patient participation in nursing care: an interpretation by Swedish registered nurses. *Journal of Clinical Nursing* 14, 1, 35–42.

Santayana, G. (1900) *Interpretations of Poetry and Religion*. New York, Harper & Brothers.

Williams, R. (2005) Professional capability: evidence- and values-based frameworks for psychiatrists and mental health services. *Current Opinion in Psychiatry* 18, 361–369.

Wilson, J. (1999) Acknowledging the expertise of patients and their organisations. *British Medical Journal* 319, 7212, 771–774.

World Health Organisation (WHO) (1978) The Alma-Ata conference on primary health care. *WHO Chronicle* 32.

PART 4
DEVELOPING SKILLS FOR THE FUTURE

12 Commissioning in health and social care

Debby Price

Introduction

The current government in the United Kingdom has been engaged in a programme of reform of the way healthcare will be provided in the UK (DH,
2004, 2005). Central to these reforms is the role of primary care and the
concept of delivering a more patient-centred service (Bramley-Harker and
Lewis, 2005). The White Paper, *Our Health, Our Care, Our Say: a new direction
for community services* (DH, 2006a) outlines the government's aim of providing
services that are designed, planned and developed around the needs of
patients. Key to the government's reforms are changes in the way health
services are commissioned. Commissioning is the process through which
organisations identify the health needs of their population and make
prioritised decisions to secure care to meet those needs within available
resources. This chapter will explore what is meant by the term commissioning
and the opportunities of this for nurses working in primary care settings.

Reforming the NHS

Healthcare in the United Kingdom has been undergoing a period of reform.
The government acknowledges that the NHS is a large and complex organisation and one solution does 'not fit all'. However, fundamental objectives for
the NHS remain and these are to:

- improve health and well-being and reduce health inequalities and
  social exclusion
- secure access to a comprehensive range of services
- improve quality, effectiveness and efficiency of services
- increase choice for patients and ensure a better experience of care
  through greater responsiveness to people's needs
- achieve best value within the resources provided (DH, 2006a).

In England, the government has implemented a 'blend' of interrelated policies and reforms to achieve these objectives. The key policies set out to achieve change and meet the government's objectives are summarised in Table 12.1.

Table 12.1 Key government policies for change

Policy	Suggested outcome
Patient choice	Patient-centred care basis of policy change. Patients are now able to choose between at least four providers including the independent sector for elective care and there are plans to increase opportunities for patients to select GPs and primary care services. The choice agenda will force providers of services to take more notice of patients' views and improve patient satisfaction
	Increased competition between providers will reduce waiting times and improve services
Payment by results	Hospitals will receive a fixed payment or tariff for each procedure. Money will follow the patient so hospitals will get a fixed payment for each patient that it treats
Commissioning and service redesign	GP practices and PCTs understand the needs of the patients they serve and will commission the most appropriate care for their patients. This will encourage service redesign and the development of patient-focused pathways to meet patient need
Plurality of providers/ contestability	Encouragement of new providers to set up and run NHS services including the private and independent sector and social enterprise. Based on theory that increased competition will be an incentive for improved cost-effective services
National targets and standards	National targets to ensure all patients will receive quality care under the NHS of a guaranteed standard and safety

Role of commissioning

The changes to the way health services are commissioned is central to the success of the government's reform agenda and will have a direct impact in the way in which primary healthcare services are organised over the next few years. For the Department of Health effective commissioning is a prerequisite for making patient choice real and the 'means by which we secure the best value for patients and taxpayers' (DH, 2006a: p3). This means:

- best quality outcomes, including reduced health inequalities
- best possible healthcare
- within the resources available to the taxpayer.

Ouvriet (1995: 18) defines the purpose of commissioning as the way to:

> [M]aximise the health of a population and minimise illness by purchasing health services and by influencing other organisations to create conditions which enhance people's health.

The terms 'commissioning', 'purchasing' and 'contracting' have been used in the NHS since the late 1980s with the introduction of the internal market. However, it can be argued that commissioning is more than purchasing and contracting in that it encompasses the following:

- assessment of health needs
- buying of services to meet those needs
- employment of a range of strategies to promote health (Ouvriet, 1995).

Commissioning, purchasing and contracting are not one and the same activity, despite the terms often being used interchangeably. Purchasing is a narrower activity concerned with buying the best-value-for-money services to achieve the maximum health gain. Contracting is simply the selection of a provider and the negotiation of an agreement to provide an appropriate quantity and quality of service. Bramley-Harker and Lewis (2005) argue that commissioning is broader than purchasing and contracting for healthcare, as the process involves planning, funding, monitoring and quality assuring services provided by healthcare bodies. Hence, commissioning is a process or cycle with key aspects of planning, purchasing and monitoring that also require the gathering and dissemination of information and effective ownership. A summary of each of the stages is outlined in Table 12.2.

Table 12.2 Key aspects of the commissioning cycle

Key aspects	Summary of activity
Planning	Identifying needs
	Determining priorities
	Understanding the market
Purchasing	Identifying providers and appropriate settings for care
	Setting contracts and incentives
Monitoring	Confirm delivery
	Reviewing quality
	Ensuring patient/client satisfaction

Primary care-led commissioning

More recently in England the shift has been towards primary care-led commissioning culminating in the drive towards practice-based commissioning outlined in the policy paper *Commissioning a Patient-led NHS* in July 2005 (DH, 2005). The term primary care-led commissioning refers to approaches to commissioning health services that involve GPs and other primary care professionals in key decision-making roles. Smith et al. (2004: 2) define primary care-led commissioning as:

> Commissioning led by primary care clinicians, particularly GPs, using their accumulated knowledge of their patients' needs and of the performance of services, together with their experience as agents for their patients and control over resources, to direct the health needs assessment, service specification and quality standard setting stages in the commissioning process in order to improve the quality and efficiency of health services used by their patients.

With practice-based commissioning, commissioning is devolved to general practice level, which can include community nurses and other allied health professionals as well as GPs. In this model, practices have the right to commission care for their patients using an 'indicative budget' allocated from their primary care trust.

The government expects universal coverage of practice-based commissioning in England by December 2008 (DH, 2005). The government believes that practice-based commissioning will result in increased patient choice, greater access to services, innovative care pathways, contestability and more involvement of frontline clinicians in influencing the types of service required and offered (Lewis and Dixon, 2005; Lewis et al., 2007; Martin et al., 2007) The White Paper *Our Health, Our Care, Our Say* (DH, 2006a: 8) argues that PBC is key to achieving improvements as it:

> [W]ill act as a driver for more responsive and innovative models of joined up support within communities, delivering better health outcomes and well-being including a focus on prevention.

Lewis et al. (2007) suggest that, more importantly, practice-based commissioning is intended to strengthen the power of commissioning relative to providers. It is suggested that strong commissioning decisions are an important counterbalance to NHS reforms such as payment by results, patient choice and the opening up of the marketplace for providers.

Practice-based commissioning is also intended to 'shift the emphasis of care from reactive treatment to proactive prevention and health promotion', particularly with patients requiring emergency care or those with long-term conditions (Lewis et al., 2007: 2) Similarly, Beenstock et al. (2006) argue that practice-based commissioning provides an opportunity to make links between preventive interventions and activity in secondary care. In the past, the connection made between prevention interventions and secondary care was limited to the extent to which redesigned pathways of care prevented demand on hospital admissions. Beenstock et al. (2006) argue that practice-based commissioning allows for an approach that moves care 'upstream'. Their argument is based on the Wanless Report (2004) that argues if prevention is taken seriously it will have an impact on demand for a range of NHS services as well as maintaining people's independence and improving their quality of life. To make a real impact on the health of local populations there needs to be a move to a commissioning strategy that seeks to prevent or delay the onset of ill health through tackling lifestyle factors such as drug use, alcohol, diet and obesity, cholesterol, blood pressure and smoking. Putting prevention centre stage and linking it to the ultimate impact of hospital activity has the potential to shift the level of debate about the NHS away from hospital beds and into the broader issues of well-being and health gain (Beenstock et al., 2006).

Engagement with practice-based commissioning has been slow and there are a number of challenges to overcome for it to be successful. These include the requirement for accurate and timely data about costs and hospital use and the need for organisational stability, which has been lacking due to PCT reorganisations. However, Lewis et al. (2007) argue that there is reason to be optimistic that practice-based commissioning will deliver at least some of the benefits identified by the government and point to evidence from reviews of earlier initiatives such as GP fundholding, which resulted in lower hospital admissions, lower prescribing costs and innovative primary and intermediate care (Lewis, 2004; Smith et al., 2004).

Commissioning opportunities for advanced primary care practitoners

The move towards primary care-led and practice-based commissioning poses a number of opportunities for primary care practitioners both as commissioners and providers of services. Martin et al. (2007) highlight new opportunities for community-based staff to develop and lead services previously not available to patients but more fundamentally illuminate the importance of clinicians engaging in the process and understanding of the national policy context. Indeed, the government has identified the desire for better clinical engagement in the commissioning process as one of the drivers for this policy direction.

It is essential, therefore, that primary care practitioners engage with commissioning to influence the process. Further, primary care-led commissioning has the potential to offer a range of exciting opportunities for practitioners to work in different ways and develop new skills. For those who want to grasp the opportunity, it will potentially allow practitioners to:

- make their voice heard and make local knowledge count
- influence the range and type of services provided for their patients
- have a say in reshaping services for patients and change traditional ways of working.

So, how can primary care practitioners get involved? Obviously, this will depend on individual roles and personal choice in terms of career directions but clearly any advanced practitioner needs to have a good understanding of the commissioning process and their role and responsibilities in the process. Opportunities for involvement can be summarised as follows:

- Involvement in commissioning groups, either as members or attending forums, to keep informed and to contribute to the planning and feedback of services. As previously stated, clinical involvement is key to successful commissioning.
- Contribution to the analysis of health needs in local area – community practitioners are crucial to the collection of informed local knowledge about health needs.
- Ensuring you have a thorough knowledge of changes happening in your local area, so that you can make sure that patients and colleagues are aware of new services.
- Development of new skills such as those needed for caring for patients with long-term conditions, community profiling and health needs assessment and business skills to enable them to set up new services.
- For some, primary care-led commissioning will provide exciting business opportunities including nurse partnerships or setting up social enterprise projects (see Chapter 13).

Crucial to getting involved and participating effectively is a good understanding of the different elements of the commissioning cycle. The cycle will now be explored in more depth.

The commissioning cycle

A number of different models of the commissioning cycle have been proposed (Bramley-Harker and Lewis 2005; DH 2006b) but in essence they all contain the same key elements. A diagram illustrating the key stages of the commissioning cycle is shown in Figure 12.1. The purpose of the commissioning cycle is to identify the steps needed to ensure effective commissioning. It describes the main stages of the commissioning process and the tasks to be addressed within each stage. For effective commissioning to be achieved there needs to be success in all the stages of the process and as with any cyclical process tasks are interlinked. At the centre of any commissioning cycle must be the needs of the service user and the emphasis of designing services around them (DH, 2006b).

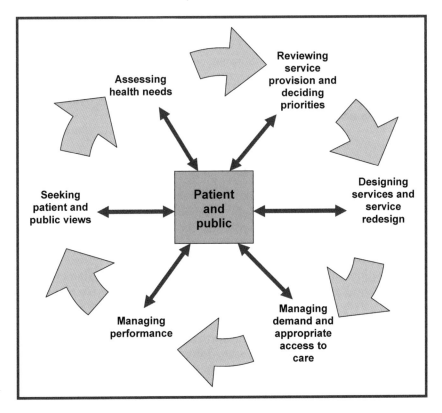

Figure 12.1 Commissioning cycle (adapted from DH, 2006b)

Each element of the cycle will now be outlined and the potential role of the advanced primary care practitioner identified.

Assessing health needs

Health needs assessment is the first step of the commissioning process and is the most effective method to determine the health needs of communities.

It is a systematic method for reviewing the health issues facing a population, leading to agreed priorities and resource allocation that will improve health and reduce inequalities. Local data, health or caseload profiling with activity data can be used, with particular emphasis on health outcomes and key achievements. Increasingly, information gathered will be based on more rigorous analytical approaches including population segmentation and risk stratification. However, the process will be a team approach and involve public health practitioners, local authorities, general practitioners, primary care nurses and other health professionals, patients and the local community (see *Box 12.1*).

Box 12.1 Primary care practitioner involvement 1

The majority of primary care practitioners have invaluable local knowledge of health need within their locality, caseload or practice and clearly have a contribution to make to this stage of the process.

Reviewing service provision and deciding priorities

This activity is clearly linked to the assessment of health needs and requires PCTs, general practices, primary care nurses and other health professionals to identify gaps in services and the potential for improvements in existing services. It is essential to seek out patients and public views on current service provision to help identify any gaps. Part of this exercise will be an evaluation of how national targets are being met (e.g. national service frameworks or NICE guidance). It is the PCT's responsibility to pull together the intelligence gained to clearly identify gaps in service provision and broader requirements for service development.

From this, the PCT will produce a strategic plan for the health of its community, which will define how the future health services will be configured, how they may differ from current arrangements and identify clearly defined milestones and key priorities. The PCT will need to work in close conjunction with general practices, patients and the local community in the process of identifying priorities. This plan will clearly signal commissioning priorities and the needs and opportunities to service providers (see *Box 12.2*).

> **Box 12.2** Primary care practitioner involvement 2
>
> Primary care practitioners have good intelligence about gaps in services for their patients and clients and suggestions for improvements to services and areas which need to be prioritised.

Designing services and service redesign

General practices including primary care nurses will work in consortias to develop strategies including new service models and patient care pathways to meet identified priorities, unmet needs and improve the healthcare of the local population. A key driver of commissioning a patient-led NHS (DH, 2005) is the government's strategy to develop healthcare outside hospitals and, where possible, relocate services in the community and primary care. This is providing opportunities for the private and third sector. Resources must be used creatively to add value and services must be developed in the right place, at the right time, provided by the right people (see *Box 12.3*).

> **Box 12.3** Primary care practitioner involvement 3
>
> Here, primary care practitioners have the opportunity to think through the best models and providers to provide care for their clients/patients and identify new, innovative approaches to improve the delivery of care.
>
> Some groups of entrepreneurial practitioners may identify opportunities to develop new provider models and set up their own business or social enterprise to provide services to meet new priorities.

Managing demand and appropriate access to care

PCTs and general practices will establish strategies to ensure patients receive the most appropriate care in the right setting and to ensure that available healthcare resource is maximised. Key to this is the role of individual practitioners in assessing patients, making referrals and advising patients on choices available to them. The importance of integrated working between PCTs, general practices, social services and the third sector is vital to ensure the best use of resources (see *Box 12.4*).

> **Box 12.4** Primary care practitioner involvement 4
>
> It is essential primary care practitioners are fully informed of options available for their patients, to facilitate patient choice and ensure most appropriate use of available healthcare resources to benefit their patients.

Managing performance

Crucial to effective commissioning is clear monitoring of the services patients receive and ensuring PCTs and general practices achieve value for money and financial balance. Systems need to be developed to allow clear monitoring of services provided through accurate, relevant and timely data (DH, 2006) (see *Box 12.5*).

Box 12.5 Primary care practitioner involvement 5

Primary care practitioners are ideally placed to seek out the views of their patients and to encourage them to take part in user/patient satisfaction surveys or user groups or forums.

Seeking patient and public views

As already stated the experience of the patient is at the centre of the commissioning process and part of this is finding out patients' views of the care they have received. PCTs and general practices will be responsible for collecting information about patients' views and experiences and to monitor patient satisfaction. This will be used to inform decisions about design of current services and future proprieties (see *Box 12.6*).

Box 12.6 Primary care practitioner involvement 6

Primary care practitioners are in a 'frontline position' to monitor and report back on the quality and effectiveness of the services their patients are receiving.

In conclusion, the discussion of the commissioning cycle clearly identifies potential areas in which advanced primary care practitioners can get involved at every stage of the process. Primary care nurses should not leave this arena to the PCT commissioners and their GP colleagues as they clearly have a vital role to play. Two key areas will now be discussed in more detail:

- assessing health needs
- new provider models.

Assessing health needs

The assessment of health needs of a chosen community or practice population is a crucial first step in the commissioning process and one in which primary care nurses have an important role to play. The outcome of the needs assessment is to create a profile of the local area and begin the process of identifying priorities and preferred patterns of service delivery and to support the decisions made by the commissioners.

As already identified, one of the objectives of commissioning is to achieve the best quality outcomes including a reduction of inequalities in health. The just distribution of health resources has long been a key principle of the NHS (Baker, 2003). *Choosing Health* (DH, 2004) places an emphasis on prevention and early interventions which can be cost effective in reducing longer-term ill health. Commissioners and providers need to stay abreast of national initiatives to improve the quality of health and social care where these may impact on health services.

Commissioners will also need clinical expertise to underpin and inform the decision-making process. For example, practitioners will be able to advise about population needs and offer advice on how services can be delivered. Some practitioners working in the community are familiar with the concept of health needs assessment as it is a fundamental part of their role (e.g. specialist public health nurses) but all are able to contribute to the gathering of health information to inform the commissioning process. An understanding of the process of health needs assessment is therefore relevant to all primary care practitioners involved in commissioning. The public health team within the PCT will also be able to provide professional advice and support to providers when searching for health needs, analysis of data for trends and demographics. The annual public health report will also contain relevant and useful information and statistics, which should inform service planning and delivery.

The Health Development Agency (HDA) defined health needs assessment as a systematic method for reviewing the health issues facing a population, leading to agreed priorities and resource allocation to improve health and reduce inequalities (HDA, 2005).

A good health needs assessment will use information gathered from a range of sources. Epidemiological and statistical data are clearly essential but the government expectations are that patients and clients should be at the centre of the commissioning process and therefore their views and perceptions must be sought at this stage. Key sources of information are now identified.

Epidemiological data

Public health departments are key to providing local epidemiological information including mortality, morbidity and loss of social functioning statistics. These provide a good starting point in providing information on death rates, level of ill health present in a given population and fertility rates.

Statistical data is popular as it is quantitative information and can be used to make comparisons with other areas or with national statistics.

However, epidemiology is a blunt instrument and the impact of statistics is reduced if used in isolation from other sources of information (Chase and Davies, 1991; Cowley, 2002). As Cowley (2002) points out, epidemiological data can provide a comprehensive picture of health need in some populations, but is unable to provide experiential information about stresses of everyday life that may lead to ill health.

Another tool used when interrogating epidemiological data is indicators of deprivation, for example, Jarman's (1984) score. While these have some merit they can give a distorted picture and may mask areas of acute deprivation within an otherwise affluent area.

Another issue with using epidemiological data in isolation is that groups of people maybe stereotyped as 'in need' while their own perceptions are different. For example, lone parents are regularly identified as being 'in need' but individual lone parents may have a different perception (Cowley, 2002).

Client/patient views

Public consultation both with individual patients and with user groups is seen as a vital area in the commissioning cycle and is essential in the identification of health needs within a community. A range of different strategies can be used to seek the views of patients, consumers and user groups including client feedback forums, public meetings, user groups and satisfaction surveys. In addition, focus groups have been seen as a valuable method to explore patients' perceptions of need.

Finding out the views and perceptions of patients and clients are not without problems. A key weakness is the reliability of the sample of patients consulted (Cowley, 2002). It is important that tools developed guard against the tendency for the more articulate consumer voice to be heard the loudest and inadvertently reinforce the inequalities in service provision rather than addressing it (Rodgers, 1994).

Cowley (2002) highlights the importance of the role of community nurses in helping to gather the views and perceptions of patients and clients. Community nurses are well placed to participate in the development of meaningful consumer satisfaction surveys and ensuring representative participation in consultation procedures.

The HDA (2005) identified five key steps in the health needs assessment process which, while not directly applicable to the commissioning cycle, are useful in thinking about getting involved in analysing health need. These steps are of particular use if you are involved in identifying the health need of a particular population within your PCT or general practice to contribute towards the overall assessment. The five stages are:

1   **Getting started:** by the end of this step the population group being assessed will be clearly defined (for example, it could be patients with diabetes in a GP practice population or families with children under 4 in a defined geographical location). There will be a clear rationale as to why this population is being assessed, who should be involved (professionals and consumers) and where the key sources of information are.

2   **Identifying health priorities:** this stage involves the identification of factors and conditions that may have a significant impact on the health of the identified population. This information will then be used to identify key health priorities for the population to improve health and reduce inequalities in health. This stage involves gathering epidemiological data, perceptions of the population, service providers and managers and relevant local, organisational and national priorities.

3   **Assessing a health priority for action:** once the health priorities have been identified, actions need to be identified to tackle this health need. In terms of the commissioning cycle, this equates to designing services and service redesign. Key to this is the importance of identifying effective interventions to tackle the health priority and who would be best to deliver the intervention.

4   **Planning a change:** in this stage, the chosen action is clearly outlined with clear aims, objectives, indicators and targets as well as an evaluative strategy.

5   **Moving on/review:** as with the commissioning cycle, evaluation of the effectiveness of chosen actions are vital to inform future priority setting.

The process of assessing health needs is therefore an essential first step within the commissioning cycle because it is at this point priorities are set. It is a complex process in which epidemiological data and other qualitative sources of information, consumer perceptions, current service provision, national and local priorities are analysed to identify health needs for a target population. However, this results in a real dilemma for PCTs and commissioners in that they are limited in their ability to meet needs for healthcare by the scarcity of resources (Baker, 2003). Commissioners have to make tough decisions on identifying the most pressing health need. Part of this debate is identifying what is meant by fair distribution of resources. Arguably fair distribution is the distribution of resources proportional to people's needs so that those with like needs receive the same resources and those with greater needs receive more. More difficult is how we make decisions as to who is in greater need (Baker, 2003). Arguably, primary care practitioners need to be involved in this debate as they are often the ones at the frontline and most able to advocate for patients.

New provider models

Primary care-led commissioning, and particularly practice-based commissioning, will open the door for a range of new providers of community health services, providing 'contestability' or a choice of providers from which to commission services. Potential new providers include the following;

- independent or private sector
- voluntary sector
- foundation trusts
- social enterprise.

Changes in the way services are commissioned will potentially offer practitioners new and exciting opportunities to deliver services to patients in alternative ways and stimulate innovations where privately or self-employed practitioners deliver care or provide specialist services (Derrett, 2006; Martin et al., 2007). This includes nurses becoming entrepreneurs, setting themselves up as alternative private providers through social enterprise schemes. Derrett (2006) argues that many nurses will find new opportunities working with general practices that are realising their importance in developing skills and being given extra responsibilities to take on new roles, for example, managing patients with long-term health conditions, advanced diagnostic skills and prescribing, strategic leadership and even becoming practice partners.

Walsh (2005), in a strategy paper for the Department of Health, argues that the primary and community workforce will need to change to contribute in providing a more flexible and responsive primary care service. She makes the following suggestions:

- The number of primary care providers could be enlarged through the development of nursing skills and through the development of nurse-led first-contact services to increase patient access and choice.
- Extending the number of nurse-run practices and nurse partners would offer real choice to patients through increasing capacity and offering alternative models of care.
- Community-based specialist nurse teams could offer real choice to patients with long-term conditions by bringing together teams of community matrons, hospital outreach nurses, district nurses and others (Walsh, 2005).

Walsh (2005) suggests 10 potential organisational models for primary care nurses to respond to the changes within the NHS. These are summarised in *Box 12.7*.

Box 12.7 Organisational models for primary care nurses

Model 1: Nurse-run practice
In a nurse-run practice, the nurse acts as an independent contractor employing other staff (including a GP) to support them in providing a comprehensive primary care service to a registered population.

Model 2: Nurse-led primary care services
Nurse-led primary care services for specific population groups such as asylum seekers, travellers or homeless people. These groups are often poorly served by general practice and often not registered with a practice. In this model, the nurse collaborates with other health and social care professionals including a GP to provide a comprehensive range of services.

Model 3: Multidisciplinary professional partnerships
Nurses as 'partners' in multidisciplinary partnerships (as opposed to GP partnerships) would start to offer real choices to patients, both in terms of increasing capacity and offering an alternative model of practice.

Model 4: Limited companies
An increasing number of GP partnerships providing an enhanced range of services have set up a limited company to oversee this element of service. A suitably qualified nurse could become an executive director of such a company. This would offer nurses a position to influence the strategic direction of the business.

Model 5: Multi-speciality teams
Patients with long-term conditions could benefit from community-based specialist teams that bring together hospital outreach nurses, community matrons, community nurses, AHPs and physicians. The team for a particular client group or locality could hold a commissioning budget.

Model 6: Co-located nursing services
In future, nurses could be located in community facilities close to home or work such as pharmacists, children's centres or schools. This would increase patient access and offer choice of provider.

Model 7: Primary care nursing teams
Such teams could either work independently in freestanding or self-managed units or are employed by a PCT arms length provider service. Integrated and specialist nursing teams could provide services to a range of people such as housebound people, residential and nursing homes, schools and other community facilities.

Model 8: Limited liability partnership (LLP)

An LLP is a written agreement similar to a partnership agreement used in traditional professional partnerships. The difference is that this is registered at Companies House.

Model 9: Nursing cooperative

A coalition of nursing groups or practices formed around a geographical area, a client or disease group could come together to form a cooperative. The key purpose would be to coordinate and integrate primary care nursing services across an area.

Model 10: A nursing chambers

In this model, self-employed nurse consultants or nurse practitioners join a 'chamber'. Depending on the size of the 'chamber' they may also be provided with 'junior' staff support. Self-employed nurses based in such a model could provide a range of services in collaboration with hospital consultants (and others) working across organisational boundaries or solely in a community setting.

(Walsh, 2005)

It is the potential of commissioning to both increase the variety of services available to patients and to open the door to a greater number of providers providing services that are more convenient to patients and which offer innovative and entrepreneurial primary care practitioners the greatest opportunities. In the past primary care practitioners have often identified gaps in the service or ways in which a service could be improved for the benefit of their client but have had little opportunity to make changes or develop new services. Changes in the way services are being commissioned and the drive by the government to increase efficiency and patient choice will result in opportunities for nurses to develop new services either within the NHS, as a business or through social enterprise. Crucial to nurses wanting to do this is the development of their skills in analysing existing health needs and service provision, identifying gaps within current provision and the ability to make a good business case for their new proposed service. In doing this, it is important that primary care practitioners seek the views of patients, users and carers and develop working partnerships with other professional groups and see the possibilities of working with less traditional partners.

Looking to the future – broadening the scope of commissioning

In March 2007 the British government published its vision for commissioning in the future in *Commissioning Framework for Health and Well-being* (DH, 2007). The document outlines a vision, framework and practical proposals for the commissioning of services for healthcare and well-being from 2008/2009. The proposed framework builds on the aims identified in *Choosing Health: making healthy choices easier* (DH, 2004), the White Paper *Our health, Our Care, Our Say* (DH, 2006a) and in *Every Child Matters* (DfES, 2003).

Specifically, the government argues that this framework is designed to enable commissioners to achieve the following:

- a shift towards services that are sensitive to and meet individual needs and maintain independence and dignity
- a strategic reorientation towards promoting health and well-being, i.e. investing in the promotion of health to reduce the cost of treating people when they fall ill
- move towards more collaborative approaches to commissioning across health, social care and local government sectors to commission services that will achieve better health, promote inclusion and reduce inequalities (DH, 2007).

The implications for advanced primary care practitioners is the need to work closely with colleagues in other health and social care areas in developing services across sector boundaries that will both meet the needs of individuals and meet the challenge of promoting health and well-being and reducing inequalities in health.

Summary

Commissioning is being seen by the British government as being essential to achieving change within the NHS through stimulating innovation in provider services and improvements in access to care and the quality and outcomes of services provided. The government argues that clinical involvement is essential for the success of commissioning and clearly it is vital that practitioners get involved and play their part in influencing and providing quality services to meet patient need. As Dr Peter Carter, General Secretary and Chief Executive of the Royal College Nursing stated: 'The way we commission services is much too important for nurses to be invisible. So whether it is designing services or deciding priorities, assessing need or managing demand, quality of care or payment by results, nurses must be seen and we must be heard' (Snow, 2007: 13).

References

Baker, D. (2003) Primary care organisations, inequalities and equity. In Dowling, B. and Glendinning, C. (eds) *The New Primary Care: modern, dependable, successful?* Buckingham, Open University Press.

Beenstock, J., Cleary, P., Green, B., Johnstone, F., Jones, S. and Levan, E. (2006) PCT commissioning: an innovative approach. *British Journal of Health Care Management* 12, 11, 334–337.

Bramley-Harker, E. and Lewis, D. (2005) *Commissioning in the NHS: challenges and opportunities. A report for Norwich Union Healthcare.* London, NERA Economic Consulting.

Chase, H. D. and Davies, P. (1991) Calculation of the underprivileged score for a practice in inner London. *British Journal of General Practice* 41, 63–66.

Cowley, S. (2002) *Public Health in Policy and Practice.* Edinburgh, Balliere Tindall.

Derrett, C. (2006) The future of primary care nurses and health visitors. *British Medical Journal* 333, 7580, 1185–1186.

Department of Health (DH) (2004) *Choosing Health: making healthier choices easier.* London, DH.

Department of Health (DH) (2005) *Commissioning a Patient-led NHS.* London, DH.

Department of Health (DH) (2006a) *Our Health, Our Care, Our Say: a new direction for community services.* London, DH.

Department of Health (DH) (2006b) *Health Reform in England: update and commissioning framework.* London, DH.

Department of Health (DH) (2007) *Commissioning Framework for Health and Wellbeing.* London, DH.

DfES (2003) *Every Child Matters.* London: HMSO.

Health Development Agency (HDA) (2005) *Health Needs Assessment: a practical guide.* London: HDA (now available through NICE).

Jarman, D. (1984) Underprivileged areas: validation and distribution scores *British Medical Journal* 289, 1587–1592.

Lewis, R. (2004) *Practice-led Commissioning: harnessing the power of the primary care frontline* London: King's Fund.

Lewis, R., Curry, N. and Dixon, M. (2007) *Practice-based Commissioning from Good Idea to Effective Practice.* London, King's Fund.

Lewis, R. and Dixon, J. (2005) *The Future of Primary Care: meeting the challenge of the new NHS market.* London, King's Fund.

Martin, J., Black, G., Cleverdon, S., Kelly, D., Shanahan, H., Kinnair, D. et al. (2007) Developing service provision for patients in primary care. *Nursing Standard* 21, 23, 44–48.

Ouvriet, J. (1995) *Purchasing for Health.* Oxford, Oxford University Press.

Rodgers, J. (1994) Power to the people. *Health Service Journal* 104, 5395, 28–29.

Smith, J., Mays, N., Dixon, J., Goodwin, N., Lewis, R., McCelland, S. et al. (2004) *A*

Review of the Effectiveness of Primary Care-led Commissioning and its Place in the NHS. London, The Health Foundation.

Snow, T. (2007) Full steam ahead for nurses' move into commissioning role. *Nursing Standard* 21, 23, 12–13.

Walsh, N. (2005) *Developing Nursing to Transform Primary Care.* Unpublished paper for Department of Health Strategy Unit.

Wanless, D. (2004) *Securing Good Health for the Whole Population.* London, HM Treasury.

13 Social enterprise and business skills

Gill Collinson

Introduction

There is a growing interest in how the third sector in general and social enterprise in particular can respond to the public sector reform agenda. This chapter describes the changing landscape of health and social care, the role of social enterprise in shaping and delivering the new vision and explores the entrepreneurial business skills required by clinicians and managers working within this new environment.

Reform of public sector services

Creating public value is at the heart of the public sector reform agenda. The concept of public value describes the value created by government through services, laws, regulations and other actions. In a democracy, this value is ultimately defined by the public and expressed by a variety of means including lobbying, campaigning and voting for elected politicians (Moore, 1995).

The concept of public value provides a rough yardstick against which to gauge the performance of policies and public institutions, making decisions about allocating resources and selecting appropriate systems of delivery.

As a general rule, the key things that citizens value tend to fall into three categories: services, outcomes and trust. Citizens experience government policy most by using public sector services. Individual and group perceptions of these services are created from their experience of using them and the outcomes of that experience. This either inspires trust and confidence in the service, or not, depending on the person's experience.

Within the UK context a number of current reforms can best be understood as aiming to increase public value, in contrast with earlier phases of the reform agenda, which focused entirely on cost reduction. Examples within health and social care include the introduction of measures aimed at improving patient experience in the NHS and the ability to choose which hospital you wish to be referred to. The evolution of the public sector towards one that creates public value has also transformed the approaches in which they are managed (see *Table 13.1*).

Table 13.1 Evolution of approaches to public sector management.

	Traditional public management	**'New public management'**	**Public value**
Public interest	Defined by politicians/experts	Aggregation of individual preference, demonstrated by customer choice	Individual and public preferences (resulting from public deliberation)
Performance objective	Managing inputs	Managing inputs and outputs	Multiple objectives Service outputs Satisfaction outcomes Maintaining trust/ legitimacy
Preferred system for delivery	Hierarchy or self-regulating profession	Private sector or tightly defined arms' length public agency	Menu of alternatives selected pragmatically (public sector agencies, private sector, social enterprise)
Approach to public service ethos	Public sector has monopoly on service ethos, and all public bodies have it	Sceptical of public sector ethos (leads to inefficiency and empire building) – favours customer service	No one sector has a monopoly on ethos, and no one ethos always appropriate. As a valuable resource it needs to be carefully managed.
Role of public participation	Limited to voting in elections and pressure on elected representatives	Limited – apart from use of customer satisfaction surveys	Crucial – multifaceted (customers, citizens, key stakeholders)
Goal of managers	Respond to political direction	Meet agreed performance targets	Respond to citizen/ user preferences, review mandate and trust through guaranteeing quality services.

Historically, decisions regarding what was in the public interest, what services would be provided, who would provide them and in what ways, was the preserve of politicians and the self-regulating professions. More recently public sector organisations have embraced aspects of the private sector ethos by considering customer care and satisfaction; however, the decisions regarding what services are provided remain the preserve of professionals and managers.

The latest reforms, for example those outlined for healthcare in *Creating a Patient-led NHS* (2005) and subsequently in *Our Health, Our Care, Our Say: a new direction for community services* (DH, 2006a), incorporate the concept of public value, which requires public sector organisations such as PCTs to engage with users and communities to determine what services should be provided and include users in the commissioning process to determine which organisations should be commissioned to provide those services in the future.

The third sector

The government defines the third sector as 'non-governmental organisations that are values driven and which principally reinvest their surpluses to further social, environmental or cultural objectives' (HM Treasury, 2006). Included in this overarching definition are charities, voluntary and community organisations, mutuals, cooperatives and social enterprises. Such is the belief that the third sector can play a pivotal role in changing society for the better, that the government has set up the Office of the Third Sector to support and enable the growth of the third sector and in particular social enterprise.

Social enterprise

Social enterprises are businesses that have a social purpose. Well-known examples include the *Big Issue*, Café Direct and Jamie Oliver's Fifteen, but there are many thousands of smaller ventures working across a wide range of sectors including, transport, recycling and housing. Social enterprises are thought to contribute in excess of £8 billion to the gross domestic product a year (Office of the Third Sector, 2006).

The roots of social enterprise reach back to the Cooperative Movement and the Rochdale Pioneers, a group of 28 weavers and other artisans who established one of the earliest cooperatives in 1844. As the mechanisation of the Industrial Revolution was forcing more and more skilled workers into poverty, these tradesmen decided to band together to open their own store selling food items they could not otherwise afford. With lessons from prior failed attempts at cooperation in mind, they designed the now famous

Rochdale Principles and over a period of four months they struggled to pool together £1 per person for a total of £28 pounds of capital. On 21 December, 1844 they opened their store with a very meagre selection of butter, sugar, flour, oatmeal and a few candles. Within three months, they expanded their selection to include tea and tobacco and they were soon known for providing high-quality, unadulterated goods. Ten years later, the British Cooperative Movement had grown to nearly 1000 cooperatives and the principles originally developed by the pioneers are now reflected in the values and principles of many third sector organisations (see *Table 13.2*).

Table 13.2 The Rochdale Principles (1844)

Open membership
Democratic control (one man, one vote)
Distribution of surplus in proportion to trade
Payment of limited interest on capital
Political and religious neutrality
Cash trading (no credit extended)
Promotion of education

Source: http://en.Wikipedia.org

Contribution of social enterprises

The Social Enterprise Action Plan (2006) published by the Office of the Third Sector identifies four key ways in which social enterprises contribute to society, as outlined in Figure 13.1.

Social enterprises are often most successful when they tackle intractable social problems. Examples of successful social enterprises in all sectors demonstrate how they use sustainable business models to meet social need, regenerate deprived communities and employ vulnerable and often socially excluded groups.

Consumers are also increasingly demanding that companies demonstrate socially responsible trading practices and the rise in the fair trade market grew by a phenomenal 640% in the five years between 1999 and 2004 (New Economic Foundation and the Future Foundation, 2005).

Encouraging enterprise is crucial for the economic prosperity of any country. Social enterprise is part of the spectrum of enterprise that makes for a vibrant and successful economy. Social enterprises run as sustainable businesses, the only difference being that the surpluses are reinvested for social purposes rather than being distributed as dividends to shareholders (see Figure 13.2).

Finally, social enterprises are seen as an organisational model for improving what have traditionally been public sector services, including

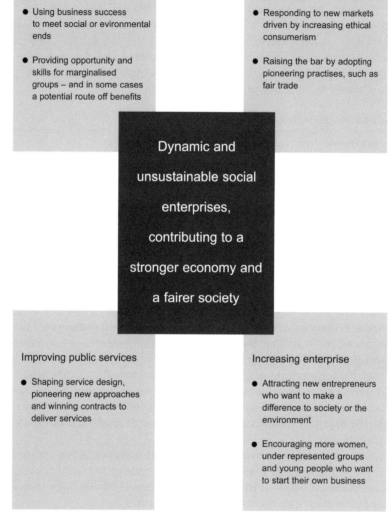

Figure 13.1 The contribution of social enterprise
Source: Office of the Third Sector, 2006

health and social care. The qualities of social enterprises that make them attractive as providers of public sector services are their high levels of innovation to solve intractable social problems and their ability to engage with users and develop relationships of trust.

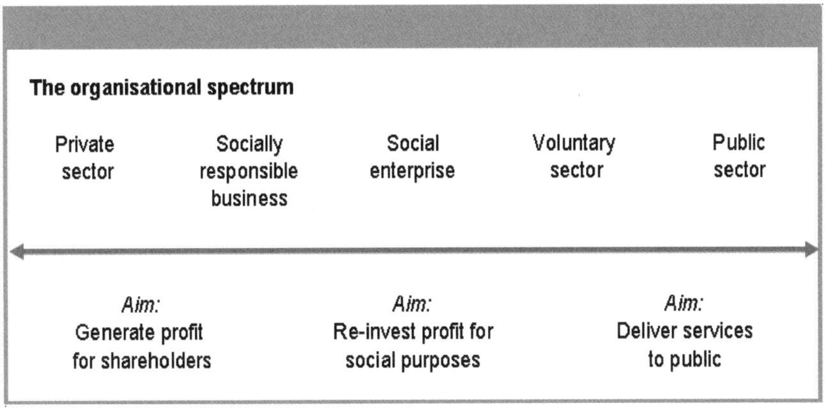

The organisational spectrum

| Private sector | Socially responsible business | Social enterprise | Voluntary sector | Public sector |

←──→

Aim:
Generate profit
for shareholders

Aim:
Re-invest profit for
social purposes

Aim:
Deliver services
to public

Figure 13.2 The organisational spectrum

Social enterprise and health and social care reform

Diversity in the provision of public sector services is seen as a key component of reforming health and social care and the concept of 'contestability' – the widening of the market to create more suppliers of services – is considered to be a key vehicle for achieving this. Organisations from across the spectrum of enterprise will be able to compete to provide services that have traditionally been part of state provision. Primary care trusts are responsible for commissioning services from a plurality of providers having taken into consideration the health needs of the population and the views of service users and the community as a whole (see Chapter 12). Assessment of the services provided will move away from inputs to outcomes, including clinical, quality and financial outcomes along with user satisfaction.

The White Paper *Our Health, Our Care, Our Say* (DH, 2006a) has four main goals: providing better prevention with earlier intervention; giving people more choice and a louder voice; doing more about tackling inequalities and improving access to community services; and providing support for people with long-term needs. It also identified social enterprise as one of the organisational business models to be developed more extensively to deliver these goals.

Development of social enterprise providers

A range of government-led initiatives have taken place to support the development of social enterprise in health and social care. The Department of Health has set up the Social Enterprise Unit to support the development of social enterprise in the sector. The pathfinder programme provides financial support and access to wider support, for example, business advice and training for 26 pathfinder projects across England. The learning from the pathfinders will be shared across health and social care, so that others can benefit from their experience and a Social Enterprise Fund is helping the pathfinders and others with set-up costs. From a policy perspective, a number of issues need to be addressed if the potential of social enterprise to deliver public sector services is to be realised.

Culture

New social enterprises are likely to emerge as a result of entrepreneurial NHS staff looking to externalise services or from existing social enterprises entering the health and social care market more fully. The cultures of each are very different and it is very important for the new organisations to consider the values and principles that will underpin the new venture and to take the very best of the public sector ethos and combine it with the business acumen of enterprise.

Risk

New ventures need to take calculated risks related to innovation and new ways of delivering services. Failures in the public sector, whether financial, organisational or clinical already exist and the management of risk, traditionally seen as a restrictive process, needs to be utilised as an enabling and supportive process.

Terms and conditions

There has been much publicity of the issues relating to pensions for potential providers of NHS services as some types of independent provider and some legal forms of organisation are not accepted into the NHS pension scheme. Imaginative short-term solutions, such as secondments, are being utilised by the early implementers of a social enterprise approach. In the longer term, however, it is clear that the majority of the workforce employed by new providers will come from the existing workforce in any given geographical area, so all issues related to employee terms and conditions, including pensions, will need to be resolved.

Commissioning social enterprises

The development of commissioning within the NHS is critical to developing the potential of the third sector as public sector service providers. The report of the Third Sector Commissioning Taskforce, *No Excuses. Embrace partnership now. Step towards change!*, published by the Department of Health (2006b) provides health and social care commissioners with guidance on how to get the best from commissioning organisations such as social enterprises.

This report identifies a number of critical barriers to effective commissioning which, if they are not addressed, will stifle innovation and the potential of social enterprises to contribute to the reform of NHS services. There is variable understanding among commissioners of what social enterprises have to offer, how they operate and their added value, that is, benefits to the community beyond provision of the contracted services. Length of contract and full cost recovery are critical issues for social enterprises, yet they are often offered contracts as short as one year, making business planning and growth impossible. An open-minded approach to the possibilities of the added value that social enterprises can bring to the healthcare economy is a critical prerequisite on the part of commissioners and they need to create a commissioning environment that will enable the third sector to flourish, if its presence in the sector is to have greater impact.

Commissioners who are innovative leaders, who know and understand the local community, the population health needs, workforce capacity and capability and clinical and organisational quality are required to ensure that services are commissioned strategically on this broad range of criteria and not just activity and price.

Limited user involvement in the planning and commissioning of services was also reported as a barrier to effective commissioning, which although relatively new, now requires a step change in the ways in which we engage with and involve users. Social enterprises are well placed to engage with hard-to-reach groups and involving them in all aspects of the organisation, including governance.

Finally, it has been argued by some commentators that the reform agenda will result in the wholesale privatisation of the NHS. However, it should be remembered that there have always been independent providers within the NHS family, such as general practitioners, dentists and pharmacists. The recently published commissioning framework (DH, 2006c) reinforces the government's commitment to the development of a diverse range of providers serving the NHS. The challenge is to ensure that the values of the NHS are evident in both how services are commissioned and provided and that high-quality clinical outcomes and user experiences determine who is commissioned to provide services.

Setting up a social enterprise

In setting up a new social enterprise, the challenges of setting up any new business will be experienced along with the specific issues of this new and emerging market.

A service or product to sell

Your business needs to sell a product or service to earn income. If it is a new service, you must have a clear vision of what it can offer.

Business and social aims

As a social enterprise, you must be able to articulate both the business and social aims of the business. The business aims will direct the way in which your business operates and the social aims will direct how you invest any surpluses the business makes to benefit society.

Market research

You need to collect evidence and information demonstrating that your business idea is viable. This step is critical and often the least well prepared, as individuals with an idea don't want to listen to the brutal facts regarding the viability of the idea. It is also critical as the assumptions made will be the basis of your business plan, which will be closely scrutinised by any potential commissioners of your service.

Legal form of organisation

People often think that the term social enterprise indicates a particular legal form of organisation. This is not the case. It is what the business does with its profits, not its legal structure that makes it a social enterprise. Anyone embarking on setting up a social enterprise will need specialist legal advice to determine the right legal structure for the specific business proposal. It is important to consider carefully the legal form of the organisation as this will have an impact on contracting and pensions, governance, finance, branding and managing risk.

Management board

The legal form of organisation you choose and the degree to which you want to create a democratised governance framework will depend on the size of your organisational membership and the number of directors who will support the strategic development of the organisation.

Business plan

The business plan tells you, your employees and all other interested stakeholders, such as potential funders and commissioners, how you will run the business. The evidence collected in your initial research will be used as a rationale for your financial projections.

Training

You will need to choose board members who bring valuable skills and experience to the management of your enterprise. Be very honest about the skills you need to acquire and use the many resources available to you in setting up your enterprise.

Start-up funding

You will need finance to pay for start-up costs, pay for equipment and provide some initial running costs. You will use your business plan to tender for contracts and apply for loans. Always try to have more than one income stream so that you are not reliant on one contract for the sustainability of your business.

Commitment

Starting any business is a major commitment and takes great energy and tenacity to be successful. Entrepreneurs have to have unwavering belief in themselves and their ideas to bring them to reality. They also have to be prepared to accept the brutal facts regarding the market, finance and their own skills in order to overcome the potential obstacles that often beset new businesses.

Developing business skills

Most clinicians have only recently, if at all, come to really consider the services they deliver as businesses. The NHS has increasingly adopted a business approach to the management and delivery of services over the past 25 years and many clinicians have made a career transition into the management of services.

However, despite this business-like approach, the very fact that the majority of services are part of the NHS means that they are in some ways protected from the uncertainties of real business and NHS managers and clinicians have not developed the full breadth of entrepreneurial skills required when contemplating starting a business.

Leadership

Any new venture needs leadership, to create a compelling vision of what might be, convey that vision to others, implement the vision, have the discipline to achieve results and develop a team to deliver the vision.

Entrepreneurs are generally very innovative and often independent, with the tenacity to bring their vision to reality. Their challenges often involve conveying the vision to others and including others in the development of the business venture. Successful social enterprises always have a leader with vision and passion but also need a team of people who are committed to bringing the vision to reality.

Marketing

The initial market research required to support the development of a business plan asks many probing questions:

- What are the trends in the market place for your particular product or service?
- Who are your customers?
- How many potential customers are there?
- Why will they want to use your service, in preference to others?
- What benefits are they looking for?
- Who are your competitors?
- What is happening in the external environment that may have an impact on your service?

Undertake a range of analyses of your proposed business including a SWOT (strengths, weaknesses, opportunities and threats) and a LEPEST analysis (legal, economic, political, environmental, social and technological factors that may affect your business plan).

Influencing skills

A key challenge for any entrepreneur is to influence others to the benefits of their business proposition. You will certainly need to influence commissioners, but there will be a wide range of stakeholders who will need to be persuaded of any number of issues arising from your business proposition. Conger (1998) identifies four essential elements of effectively persuading another:

- **credibility**, knowing your business and being considered knowledgeable in your field
- **framing a common ground**, knowing the aims and concerns of the person you are trying to persuade and creating your argument to demonstrate how your idea will benefit them
- **provide evidence**, by doing extensive market research
- **making an emotional connection**, by using stories and examples of the difference your proposal can make to those it serves.

(See Chapter 14 for further information about influencing skills.)

Negotiating skills

The skills to negotiate with commissioners, suppliers, financiers and users are critical to all those in business. Being able to negotiate price, timeframes and deadlines can make the difference between making a deficit or surplus. Surpluses mean that the social enterprise can reinvest in their social aims, so developing the confidence to negotiate and hold your ground is very important. The best approach to negotiating is to enter the dialogue with a win–win outcome as your preferred approach, but at the same time being clear as to your bottom line, i.e. the place from which, if you were to move, it would be detrimental to the business. The best way to develop negotiating skills is to practise with colleagues who are experienced at negotiating and ensuring that they challenge you in all aspects of your business, so that there are few surprises when you find yourself across the table from suppliers or commissioners.

Business planning skills

All businesses need a robust business plan that brings together where you are now, where you want to be and what you need to do to get there.

It should include a statement of the organisational purpose, vision and goals. The legal form of organisation, governance arrangements and structure should be followed by a descriptive plan of how you are going to build the business over a period of time, often 1–3 years. Financial information should also be available, along with the results of the LEPEST analysis and risk assessments.

The board must be included in the development of the plan as the directors will have formal responsibility and accountability for the performance of the organisation. Board-level discussions should highlight particular areas for review; however, the following questions are helpful to include:

- Is our organisational structure able to provide effective governance over and challenge to our business activities?
- How do we set, adjust and communicate our strategy and vision?
- Do our objectives align with the culture, behaviours and conduct of our people?
- What organisational oversight do we have at board level?
- What criteria do we set to enable us to measure and monitor performance?
- How do we govern key stakeholder relationships (public, partners, commissioners, suppliers) and communicate with them?

Networking

If you're doing it right, networking isn't something that takes lots of extra time in your life. It easily blends into your life and your approach to life. You may think of networking, making new contacts and spreading the word about yourself or your company, as attending conferences or cocktail parties to shake hands and exchange business cards.

But developing your business through networking doesn't require spending long days in exhibition halls. If you see everyone as a potential contact, you can network during any mundane daily activity. Some conversations will be fleeting, while, at other times, the people you meet will become part of your circle. Being open to staying in touch with those who cross your path is how you make your own opportunities and business contacts can come from the most unexpected sources and, at some point, you'll learn about something that can benefit you and your enterprise before the rest of the world finds out.

People tend to think of networking as going to a function but you need to realise you are building your network everywhere all the time and that successful networking is based on what you can give to a situation not what you can get.

You must know what you want from a potential contact; this sounds relatively simple, yet you must define 'want'. Be specific in your wants and look at the big picture in terms of what you can do with what you get. What you give is more important than what you want. If you attend an event with the goal of taking everything you can from everyone you meet, you won't be able to develop long-term working relationships that are mutually beneficial. A more productive way is to view this as a tremendous opportunity and yourself as an 'ambassador of goodwill', a host who is there to make sure everyone has a good time and gets what they came for. Share yourself with the people you meet and share the wealth of information you have gathered during your career in the business. If you have ideas for other people, share them. Give, give and then give again. Your efforts will come back to you in ways that are far more valuable and profitable in the long run. You will develop business relationships with people you meet at an event because you are doing something for them first and they will remember you when you call on them in the future.

Finally, be the best you can be and have fun so that you attract the kind of people you want to share in your social enterprise.

Summary

Health and social care is an emerging market for social enterprise. The degree to which its potential is developed is dependent on a number of factors not least the policy drive to develop and support it by government. Whether social enterprise becomes a major form of health and social care provider organisation or not, the health and social care sector needs more people with the entrepreneurialism, enthusiasm and determination of those prepared to start up a new business with inspiring social goals.

Developing the skills outlined in this chapter will be a prerequisite for clinicians and managers responsible for developing innovative services that serve communities and address the health needs and inequalities within a population.

Useful resources

DH social enterprise resource pack

The Social Enterprise Unit has developed a resource pack to signpost people to help and advice on social enterprise across the public sector. www.dh.gov.uk/socialenterprise

Healthy business: a guide to social enterprise in health and social care

Published by the Social Enterprise Coalition (2006), this booklet presents a range of case studies and lots of useful advice.

Keeping it legal

This takes readers through the main issues they need to consider when setting the rules and regulations that govern a business and outlines the major questions that need to be asked when developing an organisation giving information on all the legal forms available to social enterprises. Social Enterprise Coalition/Bates, Wells and Braithwaite (2006). www.social enterprise.org.uk/legal

More for your money

A guide to procuring from social enterprises for the NHS; explores how the NHS can benefit from buying goods and services from social enterprises. Social Enterprise Coalition (2006). www.socialenterprise.org.uk/procurement

Social enterprise in primary and community care

A booklet that outlines the vision of government for the role of social enterprise in health and social care. Social Enterprise Coalition (2006). www.socialenterprise.org.uk/healthandcare

Unlocking the potential

This is a guide to the different forms of non-grant finance available for social enterprises. Social Enterprise Coalition (2006). www.socialenterprise.org.uk/finance

References

Conger, J. (1998) The necessary art of persuasion. *Harvard Business Review* May/Jun, 84–95.

Department of Health (DH) (2005) *Creating a Patient-led NHS*. London, DH.

Department of Health (DH) (2006a) *Our Health, Our Care, Our Say: a new direction for community services*. London, DH.

Department of Health (DH) (2006b) *No Excuses. Embrace partnership now. Step towards change!* Report of the Third Sector Commissioning Taskforce. London, DH.

Department of Health (DH) (2006c) *Health Reform in England: update and commissioning framework*. London, DH.

HM Treasury (2006) *The Future Role of the Third Sector in the Social and Economic Regeneration: interim report*. London, HM Treasury.

Moore, M. (1995) *Creating Public Value: strategic management in government.* Boston, MA, Harvard University Press.

New Economic Foundation and the Future Foundation (2005) *The Ethical Consumerism Report.* London, Cooperative Bank.

Office of the Third Sector (2006) *Social Enterprise Action Plan. Scaling new heights.* London, HM Government.

14 Influencing and getting your message across

Rosemary Cook

Introduction

It is one of the tenets of the nursing and midwifery professions that members are expected to 'act with integrity and uphold the reputation of the profession' (NMC, 2008). In addition, those clinicians who practice at an advanced level will have knowledge, experience and insight that they want to share within their own organisations, with other professionals and with policy-makers, in order to influence and improve the care of patients and the services available to them. Both of these professional imperatives require the skilled application of the techniques of influence and communication. In more mundane matters, such as employment issues (appraisals, interviews) and professional development activities (applying for courses or bidding for project funds), the same techniques are essential to success.

This chapter aims to help the advanced primary care practitioner to acquire and practise the skills of influence in order to get their message across in any situation and a useful text to read is Cook (2006).

> **REFLECTION:** Have you ever tried to exert influence on a local, regional or national development or group? What was your experience? Can you identify what made your approach successful or unsuccessful?

Effective influencing depends on communication skills at the point of influence. But it depends just as much on the effort expended beforehand to develop the practitioner's knowledge base for influence and broaden their understanding of the issue they wish to influence. Preparation is the key to success. Following a basic nursing model familiar from clinical work, it is essential to assess the situation; to plan how to influence; to implement the plan, re-assessing and amending as necessary; and to evaluate the impact afterwards. The skills and actions linked to each of these stages is shown in Figure 14.1 and will be explored in more detail later.

It is tempting to move straight to implementation of an idea without

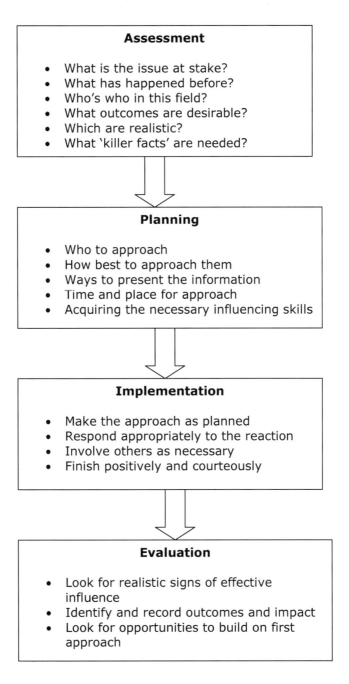

Figure 14.1 An approach to effective influencing

having completed the preparatory stages. This is usually less effective than being well prepared, armed with relevant information and addressing the right person.

Assessment: developing knowledge for influence

As a general approach, it is helpful for practitioners to take an interest in nursing matters beyond their own area of practice. It is common for nurses to read journals and attend workshops or conferences that are targeted specifically at their specialism. To broaden their knowledge, and have a better understanding of the context for their practice, it is important to take an interest in other areas. There are many topics in the news, policy, professional and educational sections of journals and conferences that apply generally across the profession. How services are organised, where the money comes from to run services and who are the leaders in the different professions or of the government of the day are all relevant. Not having this knowledge as background means that the practitioner risks trying to influence in a contextual vacuum. There are many examples of letters written to journals or questions asked at conferences that betray an embarrassing lack of knowledge of the basic infrastructure of the health service or recent developments in care. This can be avoided by making a habit of exposing oneself to more general knowledge.

Acquiring this general knowledge does not necessarily require financial resources. Many journals can be borrowed, shared or read in a library. Websites are an easily accessible source of articles, opinion, policy papers, press releases and contacts. A useful list of 'favourite' sites, to give a comprehensive round of news and views, could include the relevant specialist professional association and forum; the government departments whose policies impact on health and illness issues (not just the Department of Health, for example, but the Department of Work and Pensions, the Home Office, Department for Education and Skills and Department for Communities and Local Government); and patients' groups and charities.

Browsing this information, in web or paper form, does take time, but it is not excessive if carried out regularly and the time invested has the added benefit of adding to a practitioner's network of contacts. Names that come up as article authors, speakers at conferences, policy leads in departments or members of a special interest forum, all indicate useful people to know. An occasional email or conversation with some of them can be very useful when looking for key information as part of preparation for influencing on a specific topic.

REFLECTION: Identify an example of something you would like to influence – to improve care, develop a new role or project or change the way a policy is implemented locally. Keep this example in mind and use it to test the ideas in the next section.

Acquiring knowledge in order to influence in a specific situation requires the practitioner to shift their focus from acquiring general background to answering some specific questions. These will vary with the nature of the issue, but the following are some examples:

- What is the issue at stake? Is it really the first or most obvious issue – or is there something else behind it?
- What has happened before? It is useful to know if an issue has been tackled before and, if so, by whom and with what result. Has it been resolved elsewhere, so providing a template for success?
- Who's who in this field or locality? Knowing the local and national leaders, commentators and policymakers, at least by name, provides more people to contact for support or information.
- What outcomes are desirable? Sometimes practitioners find it difficult to articulate their desired outcome succinctly. It is useful to do so in making the approach: sometimes a simple request receives a simple, and positive, answer. It is worth spending time making the ultimate objective SMART – that is, specific, measurable, attainable and resource and time specific. Consider the difference between approaching a director to ask for 'the HCAs to have more autonomy' – which requires much more investigation and discussion and may make the director very wary – and asking for 'three HCAs with Level 3 NVQs to have a day's in-house training to be able to carry out [a specific task] unsupervised, which will save around 15 hours per week for community staff nurses'.
- Which outcomes are realistic? Ambitious outcomes are often laudable but unattainable: if major policy or service change is the goal, it is sensible to break it down into staged objectives that are SMARTer and more achievable in a reasonable timescale.
- What are the 'killer facts' needed? Knowing who needs to be approached (on the basis of having identified the real issue, sought examples and support from elsewhere and defined the desired outcomes) will often indicate what kind of facts and figures will be most effective. If the 'block' to change is the finance manager, figures showing cost of investment and potential for savings, direct or indirect, will be essential. If it is another professional group, facts

about the improved outcomes for patients may be more persuasive. For some, it will be impact on the organisation's reputation that decides their response; for others, the endorsement of a respected individual or organisation. Only by doing the background investigation can the practitioner know which levers are going to work. Networks and information gleaned from general reading will often provide the source for the key facts and figures.

With general and specific information to hand to inform an approach, the next stage in successful influencing is preparation.

Planning: different ways to exert influence

The key to making an approach as successful as possible – that is, getting a message across effectively and influencing the recipient's subsequent actions – is to choose the method that best suits the message, the aim and the audience.

The message

If it is a specific complaint, a formal grievance, a detailed idea or complex information that needs to be conveyed, a written approach is usually best. Email is probably not suitable, unless written formally and followed up by the same information in a letter. If the message is an exhortation to change, a triumphant announcement or a searing indictment, then a verbal presentation at a conference or meeting might be most effective – providing the right people are going to hear it. Using multiple media can multiply the impact: for example, making a rousing speech at a workshop session, following it up with a press release from your special interest group quoting you and then writing an article for an appropriate journal, setting out the case in more detail.

The aim

This has a strong bearing on the choice of method used to get the message across. If the aim is to express a view, positive or negative, to draw attention to an issue or to start a debate, then the method that reaches the most people and provides a way for them to respond will be most effective. Writing opinion pieces or letters for journals or newspapers, emailing a network group or 'blogging' on the web could achieve this. Contrariwise, if the aim is to persuade a specific person or organisation to implement a specific change, then a more measured approach, setting out the case in a format that is useful to the recipient, will work better. This usually means a letter, business case or meeting paper. Sometimes the aim is to point out a serious problem in practice or policy, or to highlight significant failings within a service. In this case, it is even more important to choose the most discreet method and objective language and to target the message carefully. Being criticised publicly or in front of superiors is much more likely to result in resistance and retrenchment than reaction and reform.

The audience

Targeting the message successfully, to the right people in the right way, greatly increases the impact of the message. To influence policy, contact policy officials or groups that have the ear of policy officials. They can be found through organisational websites, general search engines, the names on articles or policy documents or through network contacts (see Box 14.1 at the end of this chapter). They will need succinct summaries of the issues and proposed solutions and perhaps a couple of examples for clarification. For issues within an organisation, keep the message within the organisation, at least initially. 'Going public' before using the existing internal routes rarely achieves the desired result. Give objective facts – times, dates, names, costs, proposed actions – to named individuals or committees. If the audience is wide, such as a whole profession or patient group, the language needs to be appropriate for new entrants as well as more experienced people and the message should be conveyed simply and clearly.

Common mistakes in choosing a method to influence

- Believing that results depend on the volume or intensity of the message. In fact, quiet persuasion is often more effective than aggressive demands.
- Going on too long, verbally or in writing. Short statements have much greater impact.
- Trying to bully people into submission. This only makes people more resistant. A common mistake is copying in lots of senior people to emails. This rarely produces the desired response.
- Going public when a quiet approach would achieve results. No one likes to be embarrassed in public and organisations are very protective of their reputation.
- Taking a scattergun approach. Better to target the message carefully and only widen the audience incrementally if necessary.
- Choosing the wrong allies. A maverick who supports you may do more harm than good. Some who are willing to ally themselves – such as local members of parliament – will have their own, more important (to them) and sometimes competing agenda.

- Fighting the wrong battle. Very lofty aims and lost causes waste energy that could be better spent on a more SMART objective.

Key principles for effective influencing are that:

- less is more in most methods of communication
- passion needs to be matched by knowledge and information and the right approach for impact
- collaboration will usually achieve more than challenge
- it's always worth a second look before sending anything in writing
- battles and allies should be chosen carefully.

Skills to acquire

Writing, reading, speaking, presenting information and being effective in a meeting sound like everyday activities. But they are not always done well and, done badly, they detract unnecessarily from the impact of the message. The following pointers should act as a reminder.

Writing

Whether a letter, email or meeting paper, always aim to be brief, simple and clear. Use short sentences and short words whenever possible.

Use the layout on the page to help the reader, for example, by dividing issues using subheadings or new paragraphs. Signal decisions required or main points clearly. Do not over-use different formatting options (bold type, different fonts, boxes, shading), as this makes the page look busy and harder to read. Reread at least once before sending out a piece of writing: there is usually scope for further cutting or clearer language.

Reading

It is not necessary to do a speed-reading course, although that can be useful. For most practitioners, simply taking a more structured approach to reading will help. For example, when commenting on national policy or a local development plan, read the full document first, rather than relying on someone else's summary or coverage in a journal. Make a note of key points while reading to provide a ready-made summary for later reference. Try to read objectively, so that both good and bad points can be identified. A balanced analysis is much more impressive than 'cherry-picking' facts to suit an argument. Whatever the specific subject of the reading matter, keep the wider context in mind in order to spot unintended effects, hidden issues and potential impacts that can be used later to influence. It is useful to become familiar with the layout and structure of different kinds of document, so that it is easy to spot and analyse the relevant content. Look regularly at consultation documents, board papers, government press releases and research articles, for example, to see the different ways they present, structure and use information.

Speaking

The opportunities to influence through speaking (in settings other than formal presentations) are numerous and often unpredictable. For example, sitting next to a senior person at a meeting, asking a question at a conference or contributing to a forum discussion. So it is essential to practise, in everyday settings, the key skills of influencing through speaking. The basics include honing the delivery of your words; speaking clearly; making eye contact with the key person or the group; keeping sentences short and to the point. Marshalling thoughts before speaking where possible – for example, in a note or by rehearsing mentally – can make a big difference to the impact. Common problems that detract from the effect of the spoken word are speaking too quietly, too quickly or for too long. Making a few key points, and directing them clearly to someone, is much more effective.

Presenting information

Information, whether facts, figures, anecdotes or examples, is the foundation for influence. Without information, attempts to influence are simply a matter of one person's opinion against another's. But even the most dramatic data can lose its impact if it is presented poorly. Useful skills to acquire are:

- For figures, understanding basic statistics, putting together graphs and charts, calculating percentages, finding baseline figures for comparison, and using comparisons appropriately.
- For key facts, finding authoritative sources such as national data, research or reports for reputable bodies and from a variety of perspectives, e.g. information from patients' groups or from other industries, as well as from healthcare and the NHS.
- For patient stories and 'good practice' examples, collecting them from different sources, summarising them into succinct and effective stories and delivering them for maximum impact.

Whatever the form of information, it is also important to master the different technical skills necessary for presenting it. Skills for preparing slides and using PowerPoint projectors, videoconferencing facilities and microphones can be picked up from experienced colleagues or through training sessions. Structuring and delivering a verbal presentation for maximum impact often requires specific training, which should be regarded as an investment in a key influencing skill.

Being effective in a meeting

As with all the other skills just outlined, this is a matter of practising good habits rather than learning a new skill. People who influence effectively in meetings are those who:

- have read the minutes of the last meeting and the papers for this one
- arrive at the beginning and stay to the end
- listen to others' contributions and make their own brief notes
- contribute succinctly to build on others' points, move the discussion forward or propose solutions to problems
- give full attention to the meeting, avoiding side conversations or distractions from mobiles or handheld computers.

Implementation

A key factor in the success of any influencing activity is the way it is done. Basic courtesy, such as addressing people politely, checking that the time is right for your approach and thanking them for their time, all help to 'warm' the individual or group to the message. Conversely, a strong and well-prepared case for change or opinion will be seriously undermined if the approach is careless or impolite. It should go without saying that an aggressive approach is always inappropriate, no matter how strong the feelings or how urgent the issue. An assertive approach, however, is likely to be extremely effective. It involves:

- stating the case clearly and objectively and, if necessary, repeating it in different ways
- acknowledging others' points of view, or difficulties, in the situation
- separating the issue from the people involved and focusing on the issue
- proposing solutions or helpful next steps to move towards a solution
- avoiding accusations, blame, demands and threats, overt or implied.

At this point it is essential to be ready to handle the reaction and to take the next steps as necessary, depending on the response. It is counterproductive to take one action, then stand back and refuse to participate in the resulting debate. One action rarely has much influence: it is much more often a continued dialogue and a series of actions that enables an individual to effect change (see *Case Study 14.1*).

Case study 14.1 Continued dialogue

A nurse practitioner writes a letter to a journal on a key clinical issue. This elicits some further letters of comment from other nurses in the field, which is followed by the original writer producing an opinion piece for the journal. This leads to her setting up an email group of like-minded people, which links with a patient group to write a letter on the subject to the policy lead in the Department of Health. Two members of the group are invited to a Department of Health workshop day on the subject and take information, including facts, figures and real patients' experiences, to share. Through discussion on the day, commenting on the draft document produced afterwards, and ongoing contact with the policy lead, the nurse practitioner is able to influence the future of the key clinical issue she raised in her original letter.

Another important element of implementation is involving other people or organisations as appropriate. For example, including a patients' group, another professional or national expert adds weight and different perspectives to a case or opinion and makes it much more likely that people will listen. Defensively, involving others ensures that any flaws in the case, obscure information that could prejudice it or contrary opinions that might damage it are discovered and addressed before the issue 'goes public'.

Involving one's manager or head of department and the communications department of the organisation, similarly works in favour of an effective outcome. These people have expertise and resources that could help and, if taken by surprise by the actions of a practitioner attempting to influence change or expressing an opinion, they could react badly. Practitioners should always check whether their employer has a specific policy about permission needed for contacts or statements made outside the organisation to avoid such problems.

The final stage of implementation is the ending. Having prepared carefully and acted professionally, it is unfortunate that people who want to influence sometimes just fade away. They lose interest, become too busy or move on to another issue. By doing so passively, they leave behind an impression of carelessness that undermines all the work they have done. Some simple things that the instigator of an action can do to make a good impression at the end include:

- writing to thank people who have helped or supported the cause or action
- letting people know if he/she will not be continuing to attend a group or to lead a piece of work

- finding someone to hand over to, preferably with a written note of actions to date and any information gathered to help take the issue forward.

Evaluation

Having made the effort to put an opinion across or influence change, it is logical to look for some evidence of the difference these actions have made. Having clear and realistic objectives at the start of the action helps to make this possible, as there is a well-defined outcome to look for. Sometimes the desired outcome will be fully achieved. More often, the overall objective may take time to achieve and require the input of many people and organisations. It is still worth looking for the intermediate goals achieved through the influencing actions taken. For example, nurse prescribing from the full *British National Formulary* took many years to achieve. But nurses who responded to national consultations, wrote to the Department of Health or sat on the curriculum development group helped to keep the issue alive and contributed to practical implementation, even before the final outcome was achieved.

> **REFLECTION:** Think back to a time when you tried to achieve change or express an opinion on an issue. Did you achieve your overall objective? If not, what steps on the way to that objective did you achieve and what did you learn from it? Record these reflections in your professional portfolio.

Some ways to influence: specific points

Writing to your member of parliament (MP)

This is one way of trying to get a message into government, in order to influence health or related policy. However, it has its limitations, particularly if the MP is not in the party of government or is not an influential voice. Some useful pointers are:

- Check out the MP's biography, background, election results and previous voting record through websites (see Box 14.1 at the end of this chapter) before approaching them on a specific subject.
- Remember that MPs' principle loyalty is usually to their party and its policies – don't expect necessarily to be able to sway their opinion.
- An MP may be more likely to raise an issue with a member of the

ministerial team if approached by a number of constituents with genuine concern (not an orchestrated duplication of letters).
- When Parliament is sitting, you can write to MPs at the House of Commons; otherwise, at their constituency offices.

(For more on working with local MPs, see Campbell, 2007.)

Meeting government officials or ministers

It is surprisingly easy to arrange a meeting with an official in a government department who is working on a specific area of policy. By making an informed approach to the right person, with something of relevance and interest to their work, it is possible to interest them in further dialogue and ultimately arrange a face-to-face meeting, once it is clear you have something more to contribute. To make the first move:

- Look up which officials are working on the subject of interest, via the relevant government department website (see Box 14.1). If not directly listed, check on policy documents or consultations for the author or the named person to contact for more information.
- Email in the first instance with a well-thought out comment or suggestion, couched positively and helpfully, to elicit a response.
- Make sure you have responded to any open consultations on the subject – so as to be seen to have used the obvious channels first.
- Have a further useful offer in reserve, to be used once the dialogue is established; this could be an offer of a site visit, a paper or a good example of policy or good practice in action.

It is, of course, much more difficult to arrange a meeting with a minister. Becoming known to an official as a helpful and well-informed person on a key area of practice relevant to new policy, however, raises the chances of being invited to a meeting with a minister when such a group is sought. Writing directly to a minister may work, depending on the topic of the moment and whether your letter stands out from many making such requests. If invited to a meeting:

- Prepare as if for an oral exam – have a few, clearly stated points to contribute and be prepared to back them with evidence (headline statistics/stories rather than detailed trials).
- Examples of policy implementation or innovation in real practice are always of interest and may lead to a future ministerial visit.
- Be prepared to share the time with others and expect the minister to talk more than listen.

- Offer to send in more detailed information (which will be helpful to officials, even if the minister never reads it) rather than try to race through complex ideas in limited time.
- Expect the meeting to last for as little as 30 minutes and brace yourself for last-minute cancellations, which are not uncommon.

Using the press/media

Most practitioners instinctively understand that there are disadvantages as well as advantages to using the media to get a message across or to try to influence. Any media outlet, whether professional or general, will have its own agenda to meet. They will need to produce an angle, reflect a value set and operate in timeframes dictated by their companies. So many practitioners and healthcare organisations have had bad experiences resulting from media interest and this is often reflected by employers' policies that specifically prohibit staff other than communications professionals from having contact with the media. To avoid problems:

- Check and follow your organisation's policy on contact with the media.
- If you are allowed to communicate directly with media, ask for training, even if it is only informal training with your own communications department.
- Prepare and practise what you want to say: if speaking on the phone to a journalist, write down the three key points you want to get over before making the call. If someone calls you before you are ready, ask to phone them back in five minutes – then be sure to do so.
- Don't be afraid of journalists – treat them professionally, returning their calls even if only to say you don't want to comment. Treat their deadlines as sacrosanct – they have no choice about them. If you miss the deadline to ring back and give a comment or story, someone else will do it or the journalist will use what material they have. This may not be what you want said about your work, views or project.
- If you don't want to say that you have no comment, give them something so straightforward and uninteresting that they won't use it!
- Be prepared to explain background and not be quoted sometimes: it builds good relations with the journalist.
- Accept that you will be misquoted sometimes: unless it is very serious, it is not worth trying to put it right; they hardly ever retract or correct.
- Recognise that what you do with the media in your own time may also be seen by your employer and professional regulator. If it is

professionally unacceptable or potentially damaging to your employing organisation, you may have to face disciplinary consequences.

REFLECTION: Read the Nursing and Midwifery Council's The Code. Standards of conduct, performance and ethics. (NMC, 2008) to check its guidance on involvement with the media. How would you approach an interview with a journalist in a way that would not breach the requirements of the code?

Using the Freedom of Information Act

The Freedom of Information Act 2000 places a duty on public bodies to make information generally available to the public, unless it is of a kind specifically exempt under the act. Such exemptions include information related to policy formulation, ministerial communications, legal advice given to ministers and information easily accessible by other means. Organisations fulfil their obligations in two ways: through 'publication schemes' that make some information routinely available; and through a general right of access – providing information in response to specific requests within 20 working days – which came into force on 1 January 2005. Most public sector organisations have a designated FOI officer who handles requests for information. If seeking information to make a case or understand the background to a situation, it is worth remembering that:

- Much information is already available through organisations' websites and annual reports, which will be quicker and simpler than making a request, as well as saving public resources.
- A request does not have to be made in any specific way, e.g. by letter, and it does not have to cite the act to be treated as a FOI request.
- Requests should be as specific as possible with regard to dates and kinds of information required, to focus the searching and copying and maximise the chance of receiving useful material.
- There may be a small charge for the photocopying involved.

Summary

Advanced primary care practitioners are, by definition, experienced and committed practitioners who are likely to have a great deal to offer to the development of nursing practice and the profession. To be most effective at influencing policy, practice or change and to get a message across successfully, it is essential to take an organised approach. This involves understanding the context for the situation, planning the best approach and acquiring some specific skills, before starting out on actions aimed at influencing others. Concluding such work well and evaluating its impact is as important as starting from a position of knowledge and strength. For specific influencing actions, some useful pointers for an effective approach have been given, which will enhance the general approach advocated here and a list of useful websites can be found in *Box 14.1*.

Equipped with these skills and approaches, advanced primary care practitioners can continue to take forward their work and the expanding agenda of nursing in primary care, to the benefit of their patients, communities and colleagues.

Box 14.1 Useful websites

Nurses' professional development opportunities

www.cdna-online.org   The Community and District Nurses' Association, a specialist trade union offering employment and other support for community nurses and other primary care practitioners

www.nipec.n-i.nhs.uk   The Northern Ireland Practice and Education Council supports practice, education and performance of nurses and midwives in Northern Ireland

www.nmc-uk.org   The Nursing and Midwifery Council. For registration details, guidance on professional standards and advanced practice

www.qni.org.uk   The Queen's Nursing Institute. For funding awards for community nurses, influencing primary care policy and welfare provision for community nurses

www.qnis.org.uk   The Queen's Nursing Institute Scotland. As previous entry, but for community nurses in Scotland

www.rcn.org.uk   The Royal College of Nursing. For employment and professional support and guidance for all nurses

www.wna.org.uk   The Welsh Nursing Academy promotes excellence in nursing and healthcare through the generation, synthesis and dissemination of knowledge

Health policy

www.dh.gov.uk   The Department of Health in England

www.dhsspsni.gov.uk   The Department of Health, Social Security and Public Safety in Northern Ireland

www.kingsfund.org.uk   The King's Fund health thinktank for research and informed commentary on health policies

www.nhsalliance.org.uk   The NHS Alliance for informed briefings and commentary on primary care health policies
www.scotland.gov.uk/topics/health   The Scottish Executive health topics
www.wales.gov.uk   The Welsh Assembly Government. Follow links for health and social care

Related policies

www.communities.gov.uk   Department of Communities and Local Government. For social enterprise in health; also housing and homelessness issues
www.dfes.gov.uk   Department for Education and Skills. For children's policies
www.homeoffice.gov.uk   The Home Office. For drug and domestic violence policies

MPs' background and record

www.dodonline.co.uk   For information about the people and institutions that make up the UK parliaments and assemblies, the Civil Service and the European Union
www.TheyWorkForYou.com   For information on your MP's majority, voting record, topics of interest, etc.

References

Campbell, A. (2007) Get closure with your local MP. *Health Service Journal* 15 Feb, 26–27.

Cook, R. (2006) *Awareness and Influence in Health and Social Care*. Oxford, Radcliffe Publishing.

Nursing and midwifery council (2008) The Code. Standards of conduct, performance and ethics for nurses and midwives. London, NMC.

PART 5
FUTURE DIRECTIONS

15 The future for advanced primary care nurses

Debby Price and Rebecca Neno

Introduction

Healthcare provision has to respond constantly to changes in demographics, economics, politics, technology, patient choice and participation (Sofarelli and Brown, 1998; Callaghan, 2008). Primary healthcare in the UK is undergoing a rapid transformation as it responds to a number of key drivers including an ageing workforce, policies that demand a shift of care from hospital to community and an emphasis on prevention and care that puts the patient first and at the centre of their care.

British Prime Minister, Gordon Brown, in his 2007/2008 New Year speech to health professionals at King's College, London, outlined his vision for the NHS. He stated:

> Our goal: deeper and wider reform – building on the values, principles and idealism of the NHS to create for the next decade an NHS that is: here for all of us but personal to each of us; focused on prevention as much as cure; and strong and confident enough to put real control into the hands of individuals and their clinicians.
>
> (Brown, 2008)

He outlined three key priorities for the NHS, all of which have implications for the delivery of primary care in the next decade:

- need to embrace technological change
- need to meet rising expectations for healthcare
- need to adapt to a shift in priorities from tackling infectious disease to managing long-term conditions and 'lifestyle disease'.

Crucial to achieving this vision is the need for a flexible workforce able to work in new ways and across organisational and professional boundaries. Primary care nurses are seen as essential to achieving this.

Workforce issues

The government's strategic vision for developing and expanding primary care services (DH, 2006a) relies on the nursing workforce rising to this challenge. *Modernising Nursing Careers* (DH, 2006b) was explicit in its call for nurses to be able to work in a range of settings, to have the skills and competencies to care for older people and those with long-term conditions and be proficient in preventive and health promotion interventions. In addition, nurses need to develop both advanced clinical skills and also skills in business and strategic decision making to equip them to take on leadership roles across the health and social care sector.

Crucially, *Modernising Nursing Careers* (DH, 2006b) was clear about the need for nurses working in the acute care to develop skills in primary care. It is estimated that 4000 more practice nurses would need to be recruited in order to transfer workload from GPs to nurses (Royal College of General Practitioners, 2004), while the White Paper *Choosing Health* (DH, 2004) suggests that there would need to be an expansion of the school nursing service to meet the target of a school nursing team linked to every cluster of schools. However, this is at odds with the current workforce picture.

There are significant workforce challenges for nursing to meet this demand. Primary care has an ageing nursing workforce (nurses over 50 years of age) and will experience a significant reduction over the next decade (Storey et al., 2007). This issue has been compounded in many PCTs due to financial constraints leading to 'frozen' nursing posts and a reduction in the number of nurses accessing post-registration nursing education.

Education

Concurrently at the end of 2007 and beginning of 2008 the Nursing and Midwifery Council and the Department of Health have consecutively led consultations on the future of pre- and post-registration nursing education. Although managed separately each has a bearing on the other as a framework for post-registration education cannot be developed without considering how pre-registration education will be delivered in the future (NMC, 2007; DH, 2007a).

Wide-ranging issues were explored within the pre-registration education review all of which will have an impact for current and aspiring advanced primary care practitioners. Two of the most influential factors on the future for advanced primary care practitioners relate to the educational level of the pre-registration award with many now appearing to support a minimum educational level of degree. Where students spend the majority of their time in placement has also been consulted on with early indications strengthening the need for further time to be spent within primary care and public health settings. The current branch system (adult, child, mental health and learning disability) is also being explored, with some calls to abandon this approach. The proposals identified within the post-registration education review (DH 2007a) adopts an entirely different approach, which suggests that a framework for nursing careers should be driven by care pathways designed around client/patient need. The five pathways proposed are:

- children, family and public health
- first-contact, access and urgent care
- long-term care
- acute and critical care
- mental health and psychosocial care.

The focus of the consultation is to develop a framework that is oriented around client groups and patient pathways, highlighting the need for a more flexible approach allowing for nurses to move between pathways. The debates surrounding the future of community specialist practice awards have been abandoned until the framework for post-registration nursing careers has been identified. The Nursing and Midwifery Council has promised to address this issue once the framework has been identified.

While there are clearly challenges in overcoming education and workforce issues, the policy agenda is rapidly changing and primary care nurses will be pivotal in helping to shift the emphasis of care from hospital to more local community settings and from acute reactive care to proactive, preventive care strategies. It is suggested that the following themes illustrate the key directions for the future of primary care nursing.

Shift from care in hospitals to care in communities

This is crucial to all government policy in its desire to reform the NHS. It also reflects the Department of Health's claim that patients and clients want care closer to home or at home (DH, 2006a, 2008a) and for services to be provided at more convenient times. This will necessitate an increase in the number of health and social care professionals working within the primary care sector. New models of care based on patient pathways that dissolve the barriers between hospital and community care and between NHS, social care and care provided in the third sector must be developed. Advanced primary care clinicians and practitioners must be at the forefront in the development of such services and approaches to care delivery.

One controversial solution being suggested in London is the

development of polyclinics (NHS London, 2007). It is suggested that poly-clinics could provide the solution to bringing a wider range of quality health services over extended hours to the community, thereby reducing the need to visit hospitals and other services. It is envisaged that polyclinics would be able to provide a one-stop shop to access GP services, clinical specialists, urgent care, healthy living classes and other health professionals. Crucially, poly-clinics are being seen as a way to reduce the need for patients to attend hospital (DH, 2008). Critics of the proposals argue that polyclinics would threaten the close relationship that patients currently have with their GPs (Kmietowicz, 2007). These clinics will provide exciting opportunities for nurses to working in new settings that will command a varied and new set of knowledge and skills.

Integrated working

Essential to any new vision for primary care is the requirement for integrated working between different care agencies in order to ensure the best outcome for the patient or client. Professionals working with children and young people in children's trusts and Sure Start programmes or with patients with long-term conditions have been leading the way in integrated working. Rehal (2008) argues that integrated working reflects the fact that clients lead com-plex lives and their needs are not independent of one another and therefore care solutions must be planned coherently between health and social care services. In most cases, the cornerstone of successful integrated working is the use of a common assessment framework, co-location of integrated teams, common training, joint meetings, common referral patterns and the team being based around the patient or client (Rehal, 2008). Crucial to working in this way is for all professionals to have equal status and equally valued roles and responsibilities and a willingness to work towards a common goal. The move towards integrated working practices will become more appropriate in primary care in response to ensuring that care is patient or client focused and new care pathways and services are developed to respond to health need. The recent NHS next stage review (DH, 2008a) renews the commitment to inte-grated working starting with the support of PCTIS, we will pilot new ways of allowing primary, community and hospital clinicians and social care orga-nisations to provide more integrated services for patients including the for-mation of new integrated care organisations.

Commissioning

Stronger commissioning frameworks and decision making are central to government policy change and underpin the shift of healthcare to local communities. In December 2007 the Department of Health launched its vision for world class commissioning outlining the 11 organisational competencies that PCTs will need to achieve. In this document, they state that, 'world class commissioners are central to a self-improving NHS' (DH, 2007b: 1) and through commissioning the workforce will be motivated and fully engaged with local people and communities. The chief nursing officer has argued that nurses will have an important role to play in assessing local needs and deciding priorities (DH, 2007/2008). Chapter 12 of this book expands on this theme and highlights the importance of primary care nurses getting involved with the commissioning process.

Long-term conditions

Current health policy has emphasised the role community nurses have in managing the needs of patients with long-term conditions (Harrison and Lydon, 2008). This strategy is expected to continue and primary care nurses remain key to working closely with their patients to ensure individual needs are met and patients remain for as long as possible in their own homes. Different organisational models for managing clients with long-term conditions are rolling out in PCTs across the country. The management of long-term conditions has been further enhanced by the developments surrounding non-medical prescribing. Those who have undertaken the educational preparation for the independent prescribing programme (V300) are now able to prescribe for the whole BNF within their sphere of practice. This also now includes the inclusion of some controlled drugs. At the end of 2007 the Nursing and Midwifery Council also announced that experienced community staff nurses can now undertake a shortened prescribing education programme (V150), which, on successful completion, will allow them to prescribe from the community practitioners formulary, previously restricted to specialist community practitioners. These developments will further allow those with long-term conditions to be cared for within their own homes and exacerbations of acute illness episodes to be managed effectively and responsively. The government has further emphasised its focus on long term conditions with the commitment that by 2010, some 15 million people with long term conditions will be offered their own personalised care plans. Named lead professionals will help ensure that plans and services are tailored to support the needs of those with the most complex care needs (DH, 2008a).

Public health and health promotion

Gordon Brown highlighted an emphasis on public health and preventive health measures in his 2007/2008 New Year speech. In particular, he announced that there would be new measures to improve people's health prospects including new screening procedures for heart disease, colon cancer, breast cancer, strokes and heart disease. In addition, there would be a renewed focus on preventive care in relation to lifestyle diseases such as obesity. Following this the DH launched the cross-government strategy, *Healthy Weight, Healthy Lives* (DH, 2008b) to help everyone lead healthier lives. There are five key elements of the strategy. These are:

1 healthy growth and development of children
2 promotion of healthier food choices
3 incorporating physical activities into our lives
4 creating incentives for better health
5 personalised advice and support.

Primary care practitioners have a vital role to play in this initiative. The first phase is going to focus on the healthy growth and development of children with the target of reducing the proportion of overweight and obese children to 2000 levels by 2020. Public health nurses, midwives, health visitors and school nurses have the skills and expertise to take the lead in developing local strategies to respond to this target. The NHS Next Stage Review, our vision for primary and community care (DH, 2008a) also has a chapter dedicated to promoting healthy lives.

Summary

The future of primary care nursing is one of dynamic change, exciting opportunities and new career directions. The need for a creative, flexible and skilled nursing workforce is paramount. Primary care nurses will be required not only to have advanced clinical skills but also to demonstrate leadership, commissioning and business acumen. Opportunities exist across all spectra of care from public health and preventive care to caring for clients with long-term conditions and end-of-life care. Future primary care nurses could be delivering nurse-led care, developing new patient pathways or services to meet local health need, commissioning services for their patients, working in integrated teams or running their own social enterprise. Nurses could be working in GP surgeries, health centres, polyclinics, in social services or third sector or running their own businesses. The opportunities are endless and the future exciting for those who want to grasp the nettle.

References

Brown, G. (2008) *Speech on the National Health Service*. www.primeminister.gov.uk/output/page14171asp.

Callaghan, L. (2008) Advanced nursing practice: an idea whose time has come *Journal of Clinical Nursing* 17, 2, 205–213.

Department of Health (DH) (2004) *Choosing Health*. London, The Stationery Office.

Department of Health (DH) (2005) *Case Management Competencies for the Care and Management of People with Long-term Conditions*. London, The Stationery Office.

Department of Health (DH) (2006a) *Our Health, Our Care, Our Say*. London, The Stationery Office.

Department of Health (DH) (2006b) *Modernising Nursing Careers: setting the direction*. London, The Stationery Office.

Department of Health (DH) (2007a) *Towards a Framework for Post-registration Nursing Careers Consultation Document*. London, The Stationery Office.

Department of Health (DH) (2007b) *World Class Commissioning: competencies*. London: DH.

Department of Health (DH) (2007/2008) *Nurses to Help Drive World Class Commissioning*. The CNO Bulletin Issue 64 December/January, 1.

Department of Health (2008a) NHS Next Stage Review. Our vision for primary and community care. London, DH.

Department of Health (DH) (2008b) *Healthy Weight, Healthy Lives: a cross-government strategy for England*. London, The Stationery Office.

Harrison, S. and Lydon, J. (2008) Health visiting and community matrons: progress in partnership. *Community Practitioner* February, 20–22.

Kmietowicz, Z. (2007) Polyclinics are not the answer for NHS in London says BMA. *British Medical Journal* 6 October, 335, 91.

NHS London (2007) *Health Care for London: a framework for action*. London, NHS.

Nursing Midwifery Council (NMC) (2007) *The Review of Pre-registration Nursing Education*. London, NMC.

Royal College of General Practitioners (2004) *Practice Nurses, Information Sheet 19*. London, Royal College of General Practitioners.

Rehal, F. (2008) Ideology of integrated working. *Community Practitioner* 81, 2, 42–43.

Sofarelli, D. and Brown, D. (1998) The need for nursing management in uncertain times. *Journal of Nursing Management* 6, 201–207.

Storey, C., Ford, J., Cheater, F., Hurst, K: and Leese, B. (2007) Nurses working in primary and community settings in England: problems and challenges in identifying numbers. *Journal of Nursing Management* 15,8, 847–852.

Index

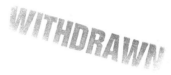